The 20% Off Diet

Abdulla J. ALkuwaiti

Table of contents

Part I - The Diet

Part II - Tools

Part I
The Diet

Chapter One
Introduction

I like to eat. I tried to look for other words to start this book, but none capture my feelings toward food in such simple terms. Food is so pleasurable because it involves a variety of our senses—smell, touch, taste and sight. Throughout the history of human civilization, we have made food, gathered around it, talked about it, written books about it, made its preparation into a profession and turned it into art. In our modern life, food has taken a new step forward with modern food technology and inventions. Food is becoming cheap and abundant, new dishes are being always invented and developed and entrepreneurs are constantly on the lookout to create that new restaurant. As I told my wife one time after enjoying lunch at a 5-star hotel: "I feel like a medieval king with all this abundance and variety."

However, food can create problems (at least for some of us). The problem is that food doesn't disappear after it passes the taste test. Because we are made from the same ingredients as food (i.e. we ourselves can be food for other creatures), we seem to mix pretty well with what we eat. So whatever we don't burn for energy gets added to our body, like excess clay on a clay man. Aside from clay men being unappealing and ugly, excess weight can cause health problems. So naturally those of us who are not blessed with "a slim body no matter what I eat" will have to work (and work hard at that) to lose the extra weight.

So the story goes like this: food is beautiful, we enjoy it, we over-consume it, we put on weight, we discover the added weight is making us less attractive to the opposite sex and we start having nightmares about the possibility of using a needle to inject insulin everyday. We decide to lose weight. We can do it (it is "we" who added the weight, and "we" who will remove it). We log on to the Internet and read about nutrition and calories, we start a diet, we buy a membership to the health club and then we get back to our prior weight. The weight is gone, very simple. Unfortunately, the last part of the story is not exactly true. I mean, the part with the happy ending. The "realistic" last part usually goes like this: we decide to lose weight, we start a diet, and we begin in the morning and quit before dinner. We go on another diet, but we quit because we are invited to a wedding party. We then start yet another diet, but we postpone it till after the holiday season. We get smarter, read books and discover that food has those tiny things called calories that we need to burn. No problem. We enroll in a gym, but decide it's too far from home. We buy an exercise machine, but it doesn't feel as good as the ones in the gym, so it becomes an expensive clothes hanger. We have another great idea. We buy $200 running shoes, a $100 shirt, a $100 pair of pants and an iPod (running in style is important). We run the first day, but the next day it's raining. We have nothing to do, so we watch TV and see a commercial for a new exercise machine. We call the store and go buy it, but postpone exercising till the machine arrives. When it comes, we feel excited, but it's not what we expected. We read more, get smarter and become scientific-minded. We learn that there are pills to reduce weight; however, they are expensive. They are risky. Yet we still try them, and they make us miserable, so we stop taking them.

The point is there is no happy ending for many of us when it comes to losing weight. Most stories about taking off weight end with statements like "I quit," "I failed" or "My body is different from other people's." Or we use the most dangerous justification: "Life is short, enjoy it and forget about starving yourself."

In my case, I had been trying (and failing) to lose weight for 10 years. I didn't imagine that losing weight would be so difficult, especially since I had played sports during college. The need to lose weight began to haunt me. I didn't think about it every month, every week or even every day. It was so important to me that, after each meal, I literally made a promise to lose weight and made a plan to diet and exercise. Unfortunately, I found that it is easy to make unnecessary commitments when one feels full. You can even come up with your own diet, like living only on apples (which I proudly did for 2 days).

Finally, I think I have found a diet that works. It's not a gimmick, and there is no magic pill or exercise. There is no magic anything. It calls for going back to the basics, and it demands honesty and moderation.

This book is intended for hundreds of thousands of people who are trying to lose weight. It is based on my personal situation that I have shared with many people who were fit (or at least not overweight) when they finished their college years, but who gained weight with the passage of time. After I completed college, I piled on many pounds and could not figure out how to get rid of them. Read about my story and see if you can relate to it: I was fit and lifted weights during college. Losing weight wasn't even in my vocabulary (actually, I wanted to gain muscle weight). I looked at fat people with amazement: "Can't they just eat less or exercise more? How difficult is that?" I finished university, got a job, got well paid, started a family and went on with my life. I had enough money to buy new clothes when the old ones didn't fit, to eat in restaurants every day and to stuff the fridge with boxes of candy bars, juices and cakes. Actually, I had two fridges—the one with a double glass door was meant only for candy and juices. I somehow forgot about my weight. I thought the added fat was muscle, and I wasn't complaining of any health problems. Then one day, my company asked me to undergo a routine medical check-up. My doctor said my blood sugar was high and I had better reduce my weight, or I would become diabetic. Then it hit me, the harsh reality … I was becoming obese.

The thing was that I knew deep inside that I was indeed gaining weight and that it surely wasn't because of muscle weight. However, I was living in denial. I didn't know whom to blame. My conscious mind for avoiding the scales? Or my subconscious for not giving me nightmares at night about being too fat (at least I expected to have a few nightmares after I installed a full-length mirror in the bathroom)?Or should I blame my ego that gave me false confidence, that I was a sporty man and could manage to reduce my weight whenever I wanted to do so? Or my family and friends, who didn't bring up the matter about my weight quite often enough. Or did they, but I wasn't listening (my subconscious again)? Nevertheless, when I received the medical diagnostics, it was time to work on reducing my weight. I don't know if you can imagine the disappointment I felt after trying to exercise and then not losing weight. I didn't think I needed to bother about watching my intake of food. All I needed was to return to the good old days of going to the gym, but it didn't work. I felt like my body was betraying me. However, I wasn't special or different from the millions of others who are struggling to lose weight.

Needless to say, my confidence was shattered. Ten years is a long time to try to reduce weight. However, when I used this method, which I now call the "20% Off Program," magic started to happen, and the pounds finally started to go away. In this book, I want to share my experience of losing weight. I am confident that it will aid your efforts to reduce your weight because it calls for balance and moderation (with a few tricks here and there). In this book, you will find a clear framework that you can follow, different tools and techniques and some basic information about dieting to show how you can start with the program.

If I am to summarize the objectives of all human endeavors, it is to feel happy. Food is a big part of happiness. Follow this program, and you will not lose that part of happiness. On the contrary, you will live your life as it was intended, and if your age is 35, you will feel like you are indeed 35 and not 50.

Disclaimer: As in any diet program, you must seek the advice of a physician before you start this system. This book assumes you don't have a medical problem that would interfere with your efforts to lose weight.

Chapter Two
Calories

If you are really determined about losing weight, you need to know a little bit about calories. Chances are that anyone (including overweight people) will advise you to eat less and exercise more to lose weight. But what is less, and what is more? It is different for my body and your body, and unless you understand how your body interacts with different foods, you will lose valuable time trying to figure it out. Knowing about calories is simple and intuitive, and will help you to understand how your body deals with food, thus enabling you to plan what food to have or to avoid in order to achieve your target weight.

I designed the 20% Off program to be as universal as possible, and part of that is anyone can start it, even if he/she doesn't know about calories. However, the concept of calories and how your body interacts with food is so simple that you can grasp it in a few minutes. I cannot find any justification for not learning about this.

Food and Our Bodies

To understand the concept of calories, we need first to understand what is food and why our bodies need it:

- **Food**

Ever seen a marathon where runners fetch sport drinks from bystanders, take a drink and continue running? That is food. It is basically a fuel, and we need it to keep running the race of life. A calorie is the unit we use to measure that energy, just as I we use inches to measure length and pounds to measure weight. So, a car might require half a liter of petrol to cover a distance of 5 miles, and you might require 450 calorie to run the same distance.

So, food contains energy, which is measured in calories, but we must be careful since we cannot see that energy. We can feel how much a type of food weighs and see its height, width and length, but in order to know how much energy is stored in a food, we need to extract it out first. This is called transformation. It is a process similar to when you burn wood, you get energy in the form of heat and lose the wood in the process. This is important to know, i.e. to distinguish between the weight and dimensions of food and the energy stored in it. For example, a watermelon is more than a hundred times the weight of a cheddar cheese slice, but the watermelon has lower energy levels (calories) in it.

Energy stored in food is independent from the size and weight of the food. Determining how much energy is stored in food is calculated in laboratories, so you need to refer to food labels to know about that. However, after finishing this book, you will be able to make an educated guess about the amount of calories in different foods, so keep reading.

- Our Bodies

We are alive. A major sign of life is movement, and to move, we require energy. We need energy for all our activities, both internal and external. We need energy for our heart to pump blood, so we can breathe and so we can use our mind and eyes to read these lines. All humans share the need for energy to make their internal organs function, but we all have different lifestyles. Some of us have desk jobs that don't require a lot of movement, while others work in the fields. Some of us choose painting as a hobby, while others prefer sports. In addition, our age determines our energy requirements. When we are younger, we need more energy to build our bones and muscles than when we grow older.

- Putting Them Together

So, we require energy to move and function, and for us humans, energy is found in food and only in food. Therefore, I advise you to think of food as energy. It might be cruel to refer to your beloved pizza or hot fudge sundae as merely energy, but taking food back to its original purpose (which is to provide energy, independent from pleasure) should help you make more logical decisions among different foods, independent from emotions. We can summarize the relationship between food and energy by the following equation:

Food we eat in a day = Amount of energy we use in a day

If your weight is not changing, the above equation holds; however, if you are gaining weight (or have gained weight in the past), it means that you are either eating more energy (food) than you are using, or you have decreased your activities while maintaining the same level of eating. In addition, if you are losing weight, it means that you are eating less food than you need to cover the energy requirements for your daily activities, or else you are keeping your food intake as a constant while increasing your daily activities. Understanding the latter statement is a basic for a healthy weight reduction diet, which the 20% Off program will help you to achieve even without knowing it.

But why is excess food stored? And why is it stored as fat? Can't it just disappear or be stored as muscle? Well, that's how our bodies are made, and anyone interested in losing weight should work with this information to achieve the desired weight. I view it as an agreement between our bodies and us. Our end of the agreement is to provide food for our bodies, while our bodies' end is to convert food into energy. Our bodies will accept almost any quantity and variety of food that we can fit into our stomach. However, the catch is whatever food we don't use as energy gets stored as fat.

The good news is that we need energy for basically everything we do: from walking to moving our eyebrows to even sleeping! The bad news is that we don't need a lot energy to move our eyebrows. As a matter of fact, we require only about 450 calories on average to run moderately for 5 miles. Now compare that to the fact that a double cheeseburger contains almost the same number of calories. But how long does it take you to finish the cheeseburger? It will definitely take you far less time than one hour. Add the fact that a cheeseburger is more enjoyable and is cheap to buy. The last example shows that food has a more profound effect on gaining/losing weight than exercising. The effect of food was clearest to me when I got sick and my appetite vanished for a few days. I lost more weight than when I go on a vacation where I walk for many hours every day. For that reason, I designed the 20% Off program to focus more toward helping you to control your food rather than urging you to exercise more.

Food Types

Scientists have categorized food into four building blocks: protein, sugars, carbohydrates and fats. For this eating program, you need to know the following about these building blocks:

First: where can you find them

- Sugars: are mostly available in sweets (including drinks)

- Carbohydrates: are in bread, pasta and pastries

- Proteins: are in meat and some seeds

- Fats: are in oil, butter and cheese.

Second: they contain different amounts of energy, meaning that 1 gram of fat holds a different amount of energy compared to one gram of protein. Actually one gram of fat has 9 calories, and all other types (protein, carbohydrates and sugars) contain about 4 calories in each gram. Knowing this will help you choose among different food options. If you are ever in doubt about the calorie content of a piece of cheese and a piece of bread of the same size, you know that cheese is mostly fat and thus will contain more calories.

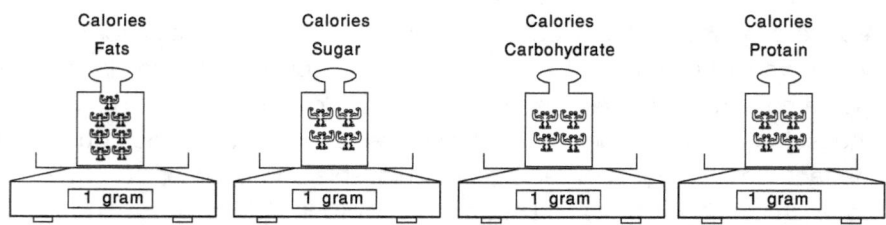

Your Energy Requirements

To use the information presented so far, you should determine the number of calories you need everyday to "function properly" and compare it with your actual consumption. Then, you should adjust your food consumption to be less than the amount of energy (calories) you use for your daily activities. By doing so, your body will start using the stored fat as energy to cover the imbalance between energy consumption and expenditure, and hence you will start losing weight.

However, in the 20% Off program, you don't need to carry a log book to write down the calorie count of every food you eat. On the contrary, the program will make it easy for you to maintain your daily routine while applying the food/energy equation mentioned above without the slightest effort from you. The program will work based on the amount and types of food you eat without urging you to change them. Nevertheless, when you advance in the program and lose much of the weight you wanted to, it will help you to use the concept of calories to compare different foods and exchange the types of food you eat for healthier ones (with lower calories) to continue losing weight. I will present more information on calories in part two of this book.

If you absolutely must know how many calories you need to consume everyday, there are different methods to find out. One famous method is using the Mifflin-St Jeor equations. Look them up on the Internet, and you will find many calculators that will compute them for you. However, if you can't wait, then most organizations approximate it to 2000 calories per day for women and 2500 calories per day for men.

There are many sources of information on calories. Search for the word on the Internet and you will get millions of results. It is not my intention to go into details about calories in this book, but to present what I believe is the most important information that has the highest potential impact on your goal of reducing your weight.

Chapter Highlights:

- Food is basically energy.

- Energy is measured in calories.

- Energy stored in food is unrelated to the size and weight of the food.

- If you eat more food than what your body needs for its activities, then it will be stored in your body as fat.

- It might not be worthwhile to try to burn all the food we eat through exercising, because it will take lots of time and effort, which is not comparable to the effort of eating

- Food is classified into 4 basic building blocks: Fats, Protein, Carbohydrates and Sugars.

Chapter Three

The 20% Off Program

Just Do It

Have you ever gone to a library to read up on a subject, found yourself overwhelmed by the amount of information available and, after thinking about which information to read, actually ended up reading nothing? How about when you decided to do that home improvement project and bought a tool kit, some books and CDs and maybe materials, but didn't actually get around to hammering a single nail? The thing with this program and other eating programs, for that matter, is you have to actually start. It is easier to spend endless hours on the Internet collecting information and watching video clips about weight-loss programs than actually to start on one. Don't get entangled in what I call the "curse of information." After finishing this chapter, you should have everything you need to start, so just do it.

Two Mainstreams for Eating Programs

There are many diet programs out there claiming to help you reduce your weight (and this book is obviously one of them). However, I want to separate these diets into the following two types:

First Type: The Breakthrough diets:

These diets promise fast results, introduce new techniques and are usually backed by big advertisement campaigns. Examples are diets that give advice on the use of one kind of food over another, or diets that claim to have found a magical seed or seaweed that will burn your fat while you sleep. Falling into the same category are diets that prescribe the use of a breakthrough gadget for exercising that promises to eliminate those "out of proportion" areas of your body.

These diets have different success rates—some are international hits and others are totally unknown. Indeed many of these diets do work, but they share a single common flaw: they all have a non-natural element in them. And that's why people don't continue with them for long. These diets don't promise or encourage a lifestyle change, but rather they encourage a new thing or way that eventually will become old and obsolete through a newer breakthrough diet.

The thing about these diets is that they work and don't work. They work in that they make us believe in them and buy their products. Yet they don't work for sustainable weight loss. The funny thing, though, is that we don't seem to complain about them if they don't work. We don't return these books or products (like exercise gadgets); instead, we just quietly forget about them and wait for the next big discovery. I think we forgive them because they gives us hope. It seems that weight reduction is a very serious matter, and we tend to appreciate anyone who tries to help us with it, even if it is with false hope.

Each year, you can expect a few diets of this type to emerge (either totally new or a modification of a dying diet in an attempt to inject life back to it), but be careful of unhealthy diets that promote the use of untested and unverified drugs.

Second Type: The Balanced Stream:

These diets are advocated by people who give advice on enjoying food but making good choices. They advise that having balanced nutrition and exercising are the key to good health. Similar to what is in this book, they call for a life change and sustainability. Think about it, you need an eating program that you can use and that will sustain you into your sixties and seventies. At that age, you will be more vulnerable to disease, and extra weight will not help you enjoy your later years.

Unfortunately, these diets don't have the appeal of the breakthrough diets. There is no breakthrough here, just the plain fact that you need either to eat less or differently. However, these eating programs need not be boring. In this book, I try to present tools and techniques to achieve the facts mentioned earlier with the least possible mental and physical effort on your part.

Now, allow me to go back to the sustainability I mentioned previously. It is very serious, and feeling the gravity of it gave me a huge incentive to reduce my weight. I knew that I was overweight. To tell the truth, I was obese (but the funny thing is, I wasn't able to use that word until I actually lost weight. It's hard to call yourself that, even if you know it's true). I knew if I didn't reduce my weight while I am young, chances are against me if I try to achieve that when I am old. I like life and want to live a long time, but I want to live a functional life. I thought that the biggest obstacle to a happy life after retirement was the extra weight, so I made up my mind to invest in my body. After all, it might be my number one "asset." Similar to feeding a few dollars to your retirement fund every month, you need to invest in a sustainable lifestyle. Start now, and you might give your knees a few extra years before you require replacement surgery due to having carried a heavy load for long time.

The 20% Off Program

This program is based on my own experience. As I mentioned in the introductory chapter, I was once slim and regularly lifted weights. However, with the passage of time and with work and family, I went from 150 pounds to more than 220 pounds. I tried really hard to reduce my weight for a total of 10 years and was always failing. I failed many times, and was about to give up. Actually I did give up many times, but the deep feeling inside me that a healthy weight is essential for my later years in life kept me trying. However, in those 10 years there was a break. It happened to me after the first 6 years, and I reduced my weight by 35 pounds in a period of 3-4 months. It happened without planning, and I didn't feel like I was on a diet at all. I didn't think much about why I was losing weight, and I wasn't following any diet program or even exercising. I was just more careful with my food choices, which is something I had tried before without success. I managed to maintain my achievement for about 6 months. I reached the state of victory. I even gave my 40-inch jeans away (I will never need those again, I told myself). You see, I became arrogant, and I felt superior to all "those" overweight people. "Can't they just stop eating so much?" I asked myself. But then it happened: I started to relax and managed to gain back the 35 pounds (plus a new 10 pounds). I tried for years to replicate that earlier achievement, but wasn't able to. I tried hard to replicate what food I had been eating and what exercises I had been doing, but with no results. It felt like a dream that I had woken out of.

Of course, not everyone who loses weight will take the trouble of writing a book about his/her experience. But it happened to me again, and after 4 years of my latest success, I am back to 165 pounds and still working on getting back to 150. My weight loss has happened like the first time, without planning and I didn't feel I was on a diet either. Unlike the first time when I managed to lose weight, I thought I must actively consider what had changed in me and why I was losing weight so effortlessly without realizing it. I thought I might have something here that is worth sharing.

Reflecting on my first successful attempt and comparing it to what I have achieved now revealed the secret that helped me to succeed. The secret was to make a proper start and maintain it for a long enough time to see some positive results. In both of my successful weight-loss attempts, I was facing difficult situations that somehow made me more determined to stick to my diet for longer periods of time. In my first attempt, I was so happy with the result that I didn't think about why it was happening or how to sustain it. In my recent attempt, however, I have the advantage of knowing that I am not immune to being overweight, and thus I have started to think actively about how to sustain my achievement. This is what led me to design the 20% Off program.

The thing that amuses me the most is, after I managed to reduce my weight for the first time and then gained it back, I was still looking for a breakthrough diet. I spent endless hours on YouTube looking at exercise equipment that, with only 10 minutes every other day, would bring my waist back to 32 inches again. I write this book to share my experience with others who gained weight for similar reasons as I did. I write it to make a record for myself—if I ever gain the weight back, I will have a reference to a program that actually worked for me. I write it to celebrate all these hours I put into learning and researching about weight loss and I write it because I used to say, "Life is short, enjoy it and don't deprive yourself of food," but now I say, "Life is short, live your true age."

My wife told me one time after I tried on a new shirt at a department store, "I didn't recognize you, I thought you were one of those high school boys." These words summed it all up for me. I had been living my life 10-15 years older and didn't know it, but now I can enjoy my true age.

The Framework

The 20% Off program has 4 elements, which are: shock yourself, don't finish your plate, use your mobile phone and reprogram your mind. In addition, the method has the following themes:

1 You need to work on your subconscious, as it is responsible for much of your food selections and eating habits. It works like an auto pilot, and will save you the trouble of thinking about each bite or sip you take. However, if you are overweight now, then most likely your subconscious is programmed to make you eat to be overweight. The word here is "programmed." You have programmed your subconscious to follow certain eating habits, either intentionally or due to outside factors like the available food selections in your environment or your friend's eating habits. Think about it: if you observe a 3-year-old boy eating, he will only eat enough to go and play, and will not ask for food again until his energy levels have dwindled. His subconscious is surely not making him overweight, at least not until he discovers French fries, chocolate and video games.

In this eating program, you need to reprogram your subconscious back to the idea of "eat to live," which we were born with, rather than "live to eat," which many of us hold as a dear motto. Now, if you are in your thirties or forties, that means you've spent many years programming your subconscious to select unhealthy food varieties and quantities. To reprogram it, you need to go slowly. It will be unfair to your subconscious to change your eating habits overnight, and it will surely fight back, which causes many people to fail in their weight loss efforts.

You will see in this program many tricks and techniques that work on your subconscious to help it to adopt new eating habits and a new perspective on food.

2 You need to keep going as long as you can without interruptions, especially at the beginning. I don't think that anyone who is overweight and is then given the chance to experience what it is like to lose 5% or 10% of his/her weight will not find a great incentive to continue on his/her

new eating program. Unfortunately, many people don't continue long enough in their programs to have that feeling, and thus quit.

Let me explain more. Turning from an overweight into a not-so-overweight person is a big change. Change indeed requires energy, but it also requires an important element, which is time. You need to stick with your program until you make some gains (i.e. losing some pounds), so it will be difficult for you to just abandon your achievements. This is just like if you take a number to be serviced by the post office. You wait for long time there, and then get tired of waiting and leave the office, and 1 minute after you leave, your number is called. Similarly, in your weight loss efforts, you need to give the program some time to work (I suggest 3 weeks). Like the example of the post office, don't quit at the beginning. Results are bound to happen.

Starting to lose weight will take time, but once it starts, the process will become easier to you. I don't have a scientific justification for the delay, but I like to think of the extra weight as ice that you need to pass through a mesh. First, you need to melt the ice, and then, once it's turned into water, you simply cannot stop it from going through the mesh. Likewise, I think you need a couple of weeks to melt that fat in order for your body to start working on reducing it. Don't be disappointed. Not many people like to wait (I am surely not one of them), but it's rather very good news that the blubber statue you have been building for years can be dismantled in a matter of weeks.

In this program, I present different techniques to help you avoid boredom with your eating program and to help you continue on the journey for enough time to see your first gains. Then weight loss will start to be exciting.

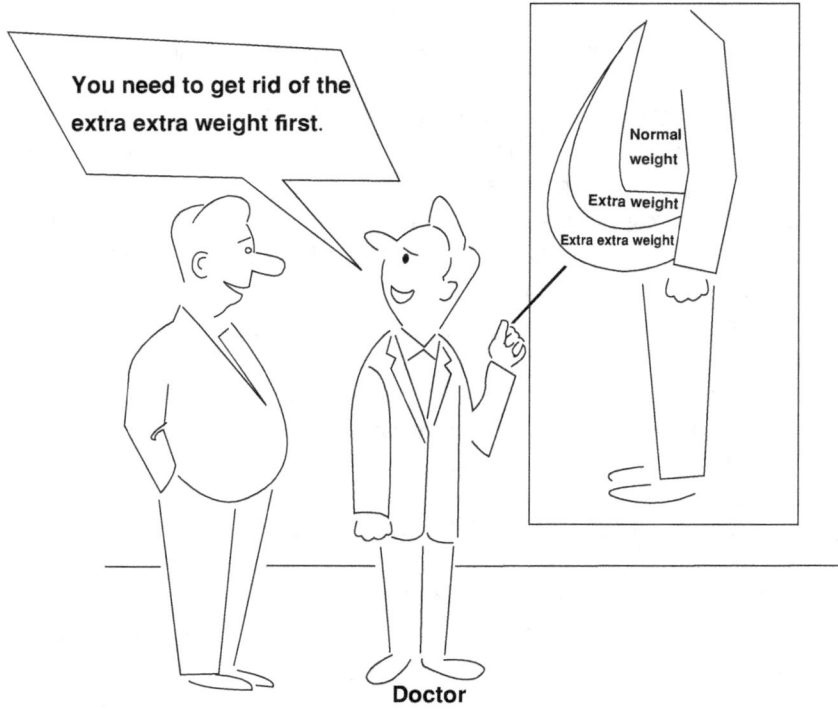

3   Honesty with yourself. I have no magic pill in this program. However, I believe it is easy to follow and won't make you feel deprived of food. I sincerely believe you can keep doing it for the rest of your life and have fun. Unlike many other programs, I work based on the truth. The truth here is that you need to balance your diet to reduce your weight. I cannot remember how many times I bought products promising an easy way to lose weight, only to be disappointed with the fine print that said, "This program must be accompanied by a balanced diet and exercise … etc." In this book, there is no fine print. All I can say is that it's not easy to reduce one's weight, but it is surely worth it.

I was overweight, looked awful and was making food decisions that would for sure interfere with my having a good life. Now, it's your turn to be honest. If you think you are in good shape while being overweight, you need to stop living in that state of denial. If you want to overeat or eat unhealthy food, you can, but be honest with yourself: you are making that decision, and it is you and only you who will experience the consequences. In time, this honesty about your health condition and food consumption pattern will feed your subconscious repeatedly until you actually make a change. If you already believe you are in good shape or immune to health problems, you will have no incentive to improve on your condition.

4 Individuality. Everyone is different. In this program, you benchmark yourself against yourself. Always try to make improvement against a previous condition you had, i.e. compare your food consumption while in the program with the past week. Compare your energy levels and perspective on food with the ones you had before.

The Elements of the 20% Off Program

First Element—Shock Yourself and Start

This is the most important element to start the 20% Off program. Remember when I told you that I started to lose weight one time without planning? It was because I had received a shock. Starting your diet with a shock is so important that if it doesn't come naturally, you might have to force it to happen. You need motivation. If you are happy about your shape and weight (or at least think you are), then you will not start reducing your weight. This is different from just seeing someone at the swimming pool and envying him/her, and then deciding to lose some weight.

You need something big, so big that it will keep the fat man inside you asleep for long time. You need the fat man to sleep long enough to allow the slim man to wake up and get stronger. When you let the slim man take control over your body for a few weeks, he will be more capable of preventing the fat man from taking over again.

Allow me to repeat what I just said, in the same way that Michael Gerber puts it in his book The E-Myth: "Everyone has a fat man and slim man inside him." If you are overweight, then the fat man will dominate your life and eating habits, but one day, when you try to lift weights and find you can't or try on your suit for special occasions and it doesn't fit, you will have a seizure. Then the slim man will be awakened, and you will start dieting. However, the seizure is usually short-term, and in a matter of days the fat man will wake up again (maybe at the sight of vanilla ice cream) and take over your body again. The thing is, the fat man grows stronger by the amount of weight you gain, whereas the slim man grows stronger by the amount of food you lose. So it is logical that if you have managed to put on weight for the last 5 years, you will find the slim man inside you very weak and unable to fight with the fat man. The trick here (which this element will help you to achieve) is to put the fat man to sleep in order to allow some time for the slim man to build some strength and be able to fight back. The longer you make the fat man sleep, the better for the slim man, and once the balance of power shifts toward the slim man, it will actually be difficult for you to gain weight back again.

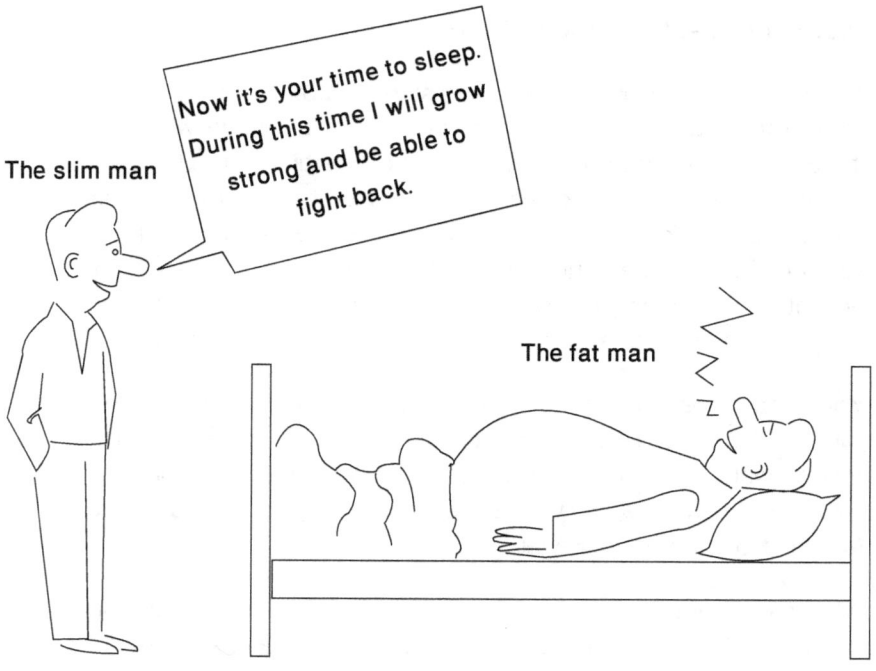

The slim man

Now it's your time to sleep. During this time I will grow strong and be able to fight back.

The fat man

Another reason why you need a shock is because, if you fall under the profile I gave in the introductory chapter (i.e. having many failed weight loss attempts in your track record), you are more likely be a procrastinator. With a shock (like the one I will explain hereafter), you will most likely start right away.

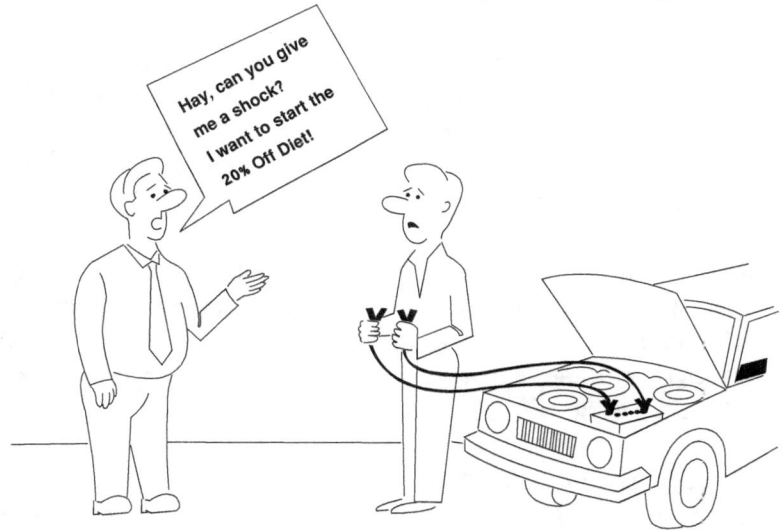

So what do I really mean by a shock? Well, it can come in different forms, but the one that happened to me and that I believe is the most effective is knowing that your health has been deteriorating with the extra weight. My "shock" story goes like this: Even as I knew that I was overweight, I was avoiding the scales, and a medical check-up was out of the question. I was obviously living in denial. My theory at the time was, if you didn't read your blood test results, your body would have no way of knowing it was in bad shape. Then finally it happened. I received a phone call from the Human Resources Department of my company telling me that I needed to update my medical records (my check-up was more than 6 months overdue—I had done that intentionally because I was afraid of being confronted with my health condition). I remember that when the nurse told me that they would take a blood sample to check, among other things, my cholesterol and sugar levels, I was hoping they would find nothing. It's like when you were young and did a bad thing, like when you took your father's notebook and doodled in it, and somehow wished that all your drawings would magically disappear and you would escape punishment. While waiting for the results, I wished and wished dearly that any high blood sugar would disappear (after all, I had fasted for 8 hours before the blood test). Unfortunately, I was forsaken by my wishful thinking. It appears that 8 hours of fasting will not undo years of using candy bars instead of toothbrushes 3-5 times a day. The doctor told me I had high blood sugar levels and that I might be on the verge of getting Type 2 diabetes. He actually gave me tablets to lower my sugar levels. Tablets! Me? No way, I told myself. "Impossible, it can't happen to me," I thought. But I knew then that my denial period had come to an end, and in a harsh but definite way.

You can imagine how I got a shock, a big shock, the kind when you say, "I didn't imagine it would ever happen to me." But I benefited from this shock. It made me conscious of my weight problem long enough to actually lose some weight and start experiencing the good life I was missing while holding onto the extra weight.

You don't need to wait for HR to set an appointment for your medical check-up. Do it yourself. Select the meanest doctor in town, the one who with a cold face who will tell you that you have high cholesterol, and when you ask him about what you should do, he will tell you to restrain your hand and put a lock on your mouth. You can also choose other shocks, like taking a photo of yourself, enlarging it and posting it on your fridge or wall. Easily said but difficult to do. It takes courage. Other shocks can come without planning, like the loss of your job or a big failure in a project (which was the shock in my second successful weight loss attempt). Try to harness these difficult situations and use them to your advantage by sticking longer to the rest of the elements that will be discussed later. You might wonder if a shock can also be positive. Personally, I didn't experience this, but I feel someone can achieve a similar commitment and momentum after positive situations, like getting a promotion at work or winning a trip to a tropical island.

There is another part to this element, which is to select a start date and announce to yourself (and others who are interested) that you have started this program. You will use this event as a benchmark to track your progress, and it should help make you more committed. It is a psychological issue that, when you declare you will do something (especially in front of people who think you are a loser), you will work harder to achieve it. However, I want you to do something that might seem unusual. That is to start the program on a weekend (preferably during a vacation or holiday) and in your most beloved restaurant or in front of your favorite home-cooked meal. This is a signal to yourself that you will continue your life as normally as you can and that you can control your food even at the places and times you associate with happiness.

Second Element: Don't Finish Your Dish

This diet was named after this element because it is at the heart of it. Do you remember your mom telling you (sometimes forcing you) to finish your dish? Now, you need to do the opposite. I am not saying not to eat, but only to not finish your food or even your drinks. Don't worry, you need to leave just a small amount of food behind in order for the program to work. For example, as a rule of thumb I recommend consuming 80% of your food and leaving the rest. So you need to leave less than a quarter of your food. Be careful here, I am not saying to put a smaller amount of food on your plate, but rather to take the SAME food serving you are used to and not eat it all. So what is the difference? you might ask. With both ways you will surely eat less.

Actually there is big difference, as big as the difference between taking and giving. When you reduce the amount of food you put on your plate, you will feel that something is taken away from you. This will introduce an element of dissatisfaction and a feeling of deprivation. On the other hand, if you put on your plate the amount of food you normally consume and then decide to leave something behind, there will be no upfront disappointment. It is you who have decided to leave that amount. Still confused? Then read along, and I hope I can convince you.

The following are some points supporting the advantages of leaving some food after you eat rather than reducing the amount of food before you eat:

1   Eyes eat: Having a full plate to start with will certainly make your eyes happier than having a reduced serving. Eyes have a direct connection to your brain, and, seeing a full plate, they will send a signal to your mind: "This is a good diet, please continue." I like to compare this strategy to the accepted wisdom that the first impression you leave on others will last a long time. Likewise, a full plate should leave a good impression on your senses. Don't underestimate the power of that perception of the amount of food in your mind. After all, it's your mind that makes you overeat, and by starting with a full plate you will calm it down, thus giving you the chance to win at the end (i.e. by leaving some food, or better said, calories, behind). Whereas if you fight with your mind from the start, by having less food, the chances are your mind will be searching for ways to compensate for that lost amount.

    Important: By a full plate, I mean the amount that you are used to eating. In your current state of being overweight, it might be one, two or five sandwiches that are on your plate. It doesn't matter, but you really need to start with your existing food requirements (while you are overweight), no matter how high they are. For example, if you are used to drinking a medium vanilla milk shake, this will be your full plate. Don't upgrade to a large milk shake and then leave 20% off it, as this will negate the idea of the diet. Remember, this eating program calls for honesty as well as individuality.

2   We are programmed to think that "more is better." I don't think I need to reference any psychological studies here. Just check your fridge and count how many items you have bought that have words like "10% more," "double the amount," "extra," etc. I mention this, as many people fail in their diet because they (i.e. the diets) are not in line with our psychology. Personally, I don't expect a diet that tells you to eat less to work for you, at least not easily. So we like more, and by following the 20% Off diet, we will be getting more (i.e. a full plate). It is true that you will get more at the beginning and leave something at the end, but it's a trick that

works, so why don't we use it? Doing so should give satisfaction to your craving for food and thus help you continue further on your program (thus achieving one of the important themes).

3   We live in a world with large food servings. Consider this story of Bill, who has just started on a weight reduction program. The program tells him to eat less food so he can lower his calorie intake. Bill follows the system perfectly at home. He might not be very happy, but at least he manages to fulfill the instructions in his diet. However, after 5 days, he takes his little daughter to a nearby shopping mall. It's lunchtime, and Bill starts looking for food. He walks into the food court and only sees food with shiny labels like "big," "jumbo" and "mega." He decides to take his daughter to a dine-in restaurant; however, he notices that they offer plates the size of car steering wheels. His daughter is very hungry by now, and he is frustrated, pressured and feels betrayed by the restaurant industry. He decides to eat that jumbo mega burger. After all, he has been dieting for only 5 days and has managed to reduce his weight by only one pound (which he thinks is not a big achievement). This decision of his is the start of his quitting his diet and going back to his previous eating habits. You may blame him. He could have just ordered a normal-size meal, but try telling that to a hungry man standing in front of cheap and abundant food.

I know it's a long story, but you get the idea that we are surrounded by a food environment where large food servings are becoming the norm. The 20% Off program will help you cope with your environment, and you will not get frustrated or disappointed by the food quantity or variety that is offered because you can eat anyplace, only you cannot finish your plate.

Based on this story, I hope you agree with me that it is more practical (and less taxing to your mind) to actually live in your environment and just take 20% off your food rather than search for smaller servings of the food you like.

4   Food is becoming cheap. So how is this related to the eating program? Well, your mind knows food is cheap and it also knows that you have

a fat wallet, so your mind (and sometimes your friends) will translate buying less as your being cheap. This will eventually put pressure on you and will lead you to think, "Why shouldn't I enjoy my food?" In the 20% Off program, you can buy your normal quantity of food and still feel in control.

5 Social pressure: Trying to eat a small serving of food can be difficult when you are around other people. It can be interpreted as being cheap or as not being able to "afford" to order a full meal. A real-life example is when I was trying to order a Happy Meal from McDonald's. It surely is smaller than a regular meal and thus has fewer calories, but I felt weird ordering a kids' meal when I had no kids with me. In addition, you might be at a party where putting less food on your plate might be interpreted as not liking the food or being angry with the hosts. Strange, but it happens. Another reason is that you might not want to be the center of attention, answering questions about why you have taken so little food. With the 20% Off program, you will have the same serving as anyone else and only have to leave a little bit of the food behind.

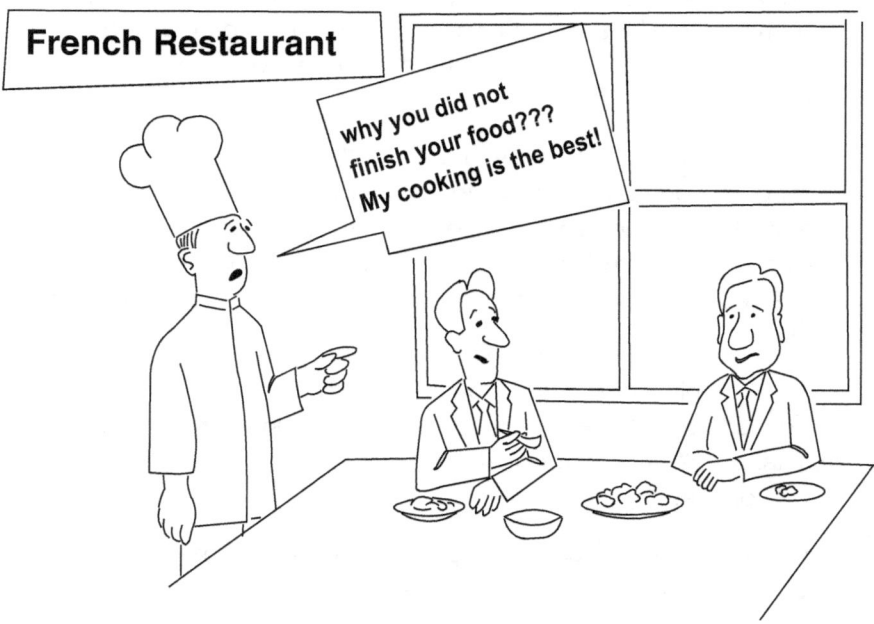

6 If you want to sustain any weight loss into your old age, you absolutely must work on your control over food cravings. If you train yourself to leave some food on your plate (while being able to consume it all), then you are in control. This is very important, because over time, you will have reprogrammed your subconscious to "eat to live" rather than "live to eat." You will develop new eating habits and will not live in a daily struggle with yourself to control your eating.

7 You don't need to worry about counting calories. If you take 20% Off your normal meals, you will be automatically reducing your calorie intake.

But why 20%? Actually it's just a percentage I feel is reasonable and will help you reduce your calorie intake in sufficient amounts, but will not leave you hungry. Also, This number works on your mind. 20% is only one-fifth of your meal, so you still have a lot to eat. You can experiment with the percentage, but 20% is a good place to start. When I first started, I was so influenced by the shock I had had that I was frequently leaving up to 40% of what I normally ate. This led me to apply another proven method of losing weight without knowing it, which was to eat more frequently over the day but in lower quantities. I tried that many times (like eating 6 meals a day), but never succeeded. Again, I attributed my failure to trying to put less food on my dish. However, when I applied this eating program, I was doing that naturally. And was seeing fast results.

I am pretty much into psychology and the connection between the mind and the body; however, I don't have scientific proof of what I will say now, but this is what I felt: When I put my normal "overweight guy" food quantity on the dish and then left some food off, I felt that my body was burning food more than it normally does. I had a feeling of a very slight burning in my stomach that wasn't painful (actually, it was somewhat pleasant). In time, I was able to associate this feeling with weight loss. When I felt it, I would tell my wife that I would weigh less the next day, and I was often right. I reasoned that when I saw a large amount of food in front of me, my mind would send signals to my stomach to be prepared to digest that amount, so that when I actually ate less, the energy available (from my stomach) to burn food was more than I needed and thus would burn food more efficiently. This, I believe, will increase metabolism and trigger a faster weight loss.

How to apply the 20% Off element

To apply this element, follow these steps:

1 You need to order the same amount of food (drinks are included in the count) you are used to ordering. For example, if you are used to eating 3 cheeseburgers at one meal, take 20% off the 3 cheeseburgers, meaning you might eat 2 and a half burgers. Don't take 4 burgers and then take off the 20%. Don't cheat.

2 Plan for the amount of food you are going to leave. Observe your meal and think of what 80% of the meal will constitute so that you know when to stop. Then enjoy your food and stop when you think you have eaten 80%. This strategy should be applied to the whole meal, including the sides and drinks. For example, if you have a meal consisting of a burger, French fries and a Coke, then leave 20% off each. There is no hard-and-fast rule here. You just need to leave some food behind. In the beginning of applying the program, take it easy and be simple; however, with time you will be able to make more creative choices. For example, you might decide to eat your full burger and a few fries. You might also order a Diet Coke instead of the normal one and drink it all.

   As long as you eat 20% of the whole meal, you are on the right track. Don't worry, I will give more examples in the next section.

3 Take it slowly. With some meals, you might have one of these strongwilled moments and be able to leave half of your meal. With another, you might only leave one bite. But leaving only one bite is nothing to sneeze at. Aside from the calories that you will save, you are building your strength against the food. That's a major achievement in its own right.

4 Don't give up. Compensate. If you finish your normal-size meal at lunch, try to compensate for it during dinner, and so on. Don't give up. You didn't gain weight from one meal, and you will not lose it by leaving one meal either.

5 Observe your achievements. After you finish eating, look at the food and deliberately think about it. Think that you could have eaten it all, but decided not to. More on that in the next section.

Note that the 20% Off program will take you into stages. Be clear on two factors: the amount of food you put on your plate, and the percentage you leave off. In your first day on the program, you will start with the same amount of food you are used to eating and leave 20% off it. In time, your body will adjust, and you will be able to leave larger amounts, up to 50% of your meals. It will be the time then to reduce the amount of the food you order and go back to leaving only 20% off (I don't want you to reach the point of ordering two burgers and throwing a whole one away). So basically, as you "outgrow" your serving size, reduce it and work to outgrow the new serving size. For example, if you can (or must) eat a dozen of chicken wings in one meal, start by leaving 3 or 4 wings behind. In time, you will be able to leave more, like 5 wings. Now you need to set a new starting point, say 8 wings, and start to leave 2 wings. Of course, this practice will not continue until you eat nothing, but rather your body will tell you when to hold your serving size. At that point, you will notice your weight loss and a feeling of satisfaction over food, but keep using this method, even if you just leave 10% off your food, because like I said, this is not a mere diet but a full eating program that will work on both your mind and body.

Obstacles in Implementing This Element:

So what's the big deal, you might think. Anybody can leave some food behind! Well, it's not that easy. For years, I was feeling full before I finished my food, but kept eating every bit on my plate (and those of my wife and kids). The following reasons were preventing me from leaving excess food when I was full. They deal with my beliefs and perception of what is right and what is wrong:

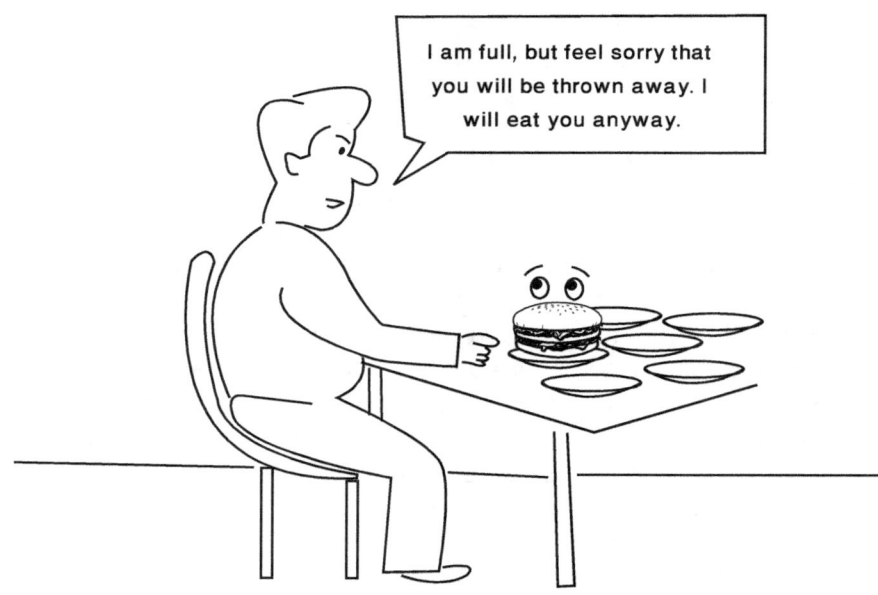

1 Leaving food behind was not in line with my beliefs, especially with overwhelming news about famine and children dying from starvation. Also, almost all religions and belief systems will tell you food is a blessing and should not be wasted. For these reasons, I was eating everything in front of me because I thought I was not doing wrong to people who don't have food (i.e. I was not throwing away anything).

2 Food is money. Not finishing your food means you are throwing money away. By finishing everything, I was avoiding blame from my friends and family that I was spoiled and wasting money.

I struggled for years between putting large amounts of food in front of me and the urge to finish it all off even if I was full. However, when I was shocked and really started to reduce my weight, my thinking started to change as follows:

1 Finishing my food even when I was full would not help poor children. If I was serious about helping them, there were other means, like making a donation and doing community service.

2 It might be correct that I might be wasting food, but I was wasting something more important: my body and my life. I thought if I continued to leave some food out, I would adjust to eating less with time and would eventually order less food. So in the long run, I would be actually saving food.

3 As for wasting money, I now think that it will cost me more money for medical bills if I am diagnosed with a disease caused by my poor eating habits.

These changes to my thinking helped me continue applying the 20% Off element and to reduce my weight and be happy. We shouldn't underestimate the strength of perception, and should dig deep into our minds to identify any obstacles preventing us from losing weight. It's easier said than done, but if you keep working on it, you will succeed.

How I Discovered This Method

So did I just stumble upon this idea? Actually, no. It took me years of thinking and observing my own behavior. I noticed the following behavior in myself: I needed to order a large amount of food. In restaurants, I was ordering enough food for two adults. At home, I was also putting large amounts of food on my plate. Even when I was full, I ordered a lot of food. For example, after just finishing lunch, if I passed by a juice shop, I would order the largest serving they had. My wife noticed this behavior, but even after constant reminders to order less, when I stood in front of the cashier, I ordered more. I wondered why I was doing that, and I think it was because of the following:

1 I like to try new food.

2 Food is cheap. It might be one of the cheapest things that will make you happy in life (certainly cheaper than a sports car). And I like to be happy.

3 I was always looking for a good deal. Restaurants and supermarkets are full of good deals: buy one get one free, supersize it for only 50 cents more and so forth. Also, when I was being asked nicely to add an apple pie, I usually agreed.

4   I liked to eat out. When eating out, I was given different options (and I liked to try different ones).

5   Like many people, I had this notion of "more is better," which translated into my life and eating habits.

6   Media influences. Like in the famous story in which a young boy and his sister stumble on a house made of cake in the forest, these media influences made me as a kid associate an abundance of food with happiness.

So, I liked to order a lot, and that is what I did. I tried hard not to do that, but I just couldn't help myself. I don't remember ever having ordered a small pizza even when I was by myself. I couldn't control ordering that extra sandwich. It was like a second nature I had developed.

After many failed attempts at ordering less food, I did a strange thing. I accepted that I needed to order large amounts of food to be satisfied. By doing so, my thinking was shifting to focus on other ways to reduce my weight. I knew that I had to consume fewer calories, so I tried low-calorie food but with no immediate weight-loss results. However, I noticed in some instances that when my eating was disrupted, I was feeling light and energetic. For example, if in the middle of my meal someone knocked on my door and I was busy talking with him for a while, I would tend to forget about my unfinished meal and I had the following feelings:

A   I was feeling light and energetic, unlike the laziness I felt after a full meal.

B   I was satisfied. I didn't feel I needed to have another meal to compensate for the incomplete one

Then it struck me that all what I needed was to not finish my food.

I believe many of you will share some of the aspects presented in this section and will relate to my story. The moral of the story is that you need to honest with yourself and identify the real causes that hinder you from losing weight. Then try to work around these hindrances, as it might be very difficult to eliminate them, but reducing their effect might be feasible and can yield good results.

Third Element: Use Your Mobile Phone

I usually dine in restaurants that offer free refills. Before I finish my drink, the waitress will bring me a full one. One time I was having lunch at a busy restaurant. The waitress kept providing me with refills, but forgot to take the old glasses from the table, so I pushed them to the side. When I was about to order another refill, my wife pointed for to me to look at the side of the table. There were two empty glasses plus the one I was about to finish. Needless to say, I felt bad for my stomach and didn't take any additional drink. The decision to pass on the additional drink was very easy to make because I could see how much I had already drunk.

I thought, what if we can always visualize how much food we actually eat? It would be easier, then, to stop overeating. The problem is, once we finish our food, it's gone, and we cannot account for it. Brian Wansink puts it very nicely in his book The Mindless Eating when he says, "Our stomachs cannot count."

Here comes the importance of documentation. It captures information for us to analyze and go back to. We can "count" the food we put in our stomach and compare it to our weight-loss results. With the 20% Off diet, you will use documentation to achieve your goal. Following are reasons for why should you document your weight-loss efforts:

1   To make sure you are following the 20% Off method (i.e. make sure you are leaving some food behind)
2   To record progress that will motivate you to continue with your new lifestyle
3   To record the types of food you are consuming and to think of better alternatives (you will need this strategy as you advance on your weight loss journey)
4   To work on your subconscious, by having evidence that you were able to leave some food behind

However, I am not here to point to the importance of documentation. You will find many studies proving that documentation will greatly help you succeed in anything you want to achieve, weight loss included. What I want to do is to present a method that will help you practice documentation. Documentation is rather difficult. It will require that you take the time and use the necessary equipment to log down what you ate at different times of the day. Actually I don't remember knowing anyone who was able to keep a log of his/her eating for more than 3 days. I tried many times and failed, even though I bought a special logbook for weight loss and an electronic organizer to log my eating. I faced the following difficulties while trying to document my food consumption:

1 I cannot take a log book everywhere I go to eat. Even if I try, I will certainly forget sometimes.

2 I felt embarrassed to write my food diaries in public places.

3 If I decide to write down what I had for dinner when I get back home, I usually cannot remember the details of everything I ate.

4 One purpose of documenting my eating is to review what food I had. However, it is boring to read what food I ate in the past few days.

5 My handwriting is not that good.

For these reasons, documentation was more of a theory than a practice. However, I found a method that will provide the benefits of documentation and is practical and actually fun. It is effective to use your mobile phone to document your food with pictures. Using the camera on a mobile phone has the following advantages:

1 Your phone is almost always with you, especially when you are out of the house. This will help you not miss recording any food you eat.

2 Even cheap mobile phones have good-quality cameras.

3 Pictures will capture all the details of your food.

4 Taking a picture of your food is much faster that writing it down.

5 You can sort your pictures by date and time taken, so you will not lose track of what you ate and when you ate it.

6   You can review your eating history in an enjoyable manner, similar to reviewing a vacation photo album.

7   A picture is worth a thousand words! Seeing pictures of food you left behind while having the ability to finish it all should work on your subconscious so that you are in control of food.

In a nutshell, your mobile phone camera is almost always available, easy to use and will save you the trouble of writing down the details. The following are examples of how to use it.

Examples:

Example 1: Applying the 20% Off to a Big Mac Meal

Let's assume you go for lunch at McDonald's: You are on the 20% Off program and have ordered your normal quantity of food, which is a two Big Mac sandwiches with a large Diet Coke.

Step One: Remember to order the normal quantity of food you are used to having.

Step Two: Observe the food in front of you and decide that you will leave 20% off of it. As an option, you can take a picture before you start eating.

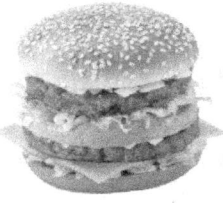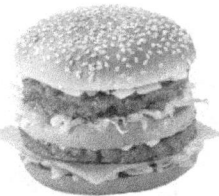

Step Three: Enjoy 80% of the food which is about one full burger and two thirds to one half of the second one.

Step Four: Stop, observe the food you left behind and feel in control because you are able to finish all your food but decided not to.

Step Five: Take a picture of the remaining food.

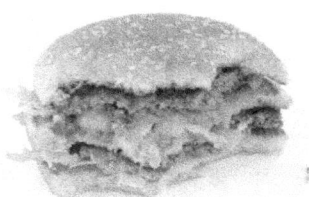

Note: if your normal order contains French Fries then you should also leave 20% Off it. As for the Diet Coke, since it might contain only1 or 2 calories you have the option of drinking it all.

Strategy in applying the 20% Off Method:

The following series of pictures will illustrate the strategy you need to adopt to make this program work. Your goal is to progress in the amount of food you leave behind, from nothing to 20% or even 50% of the food.

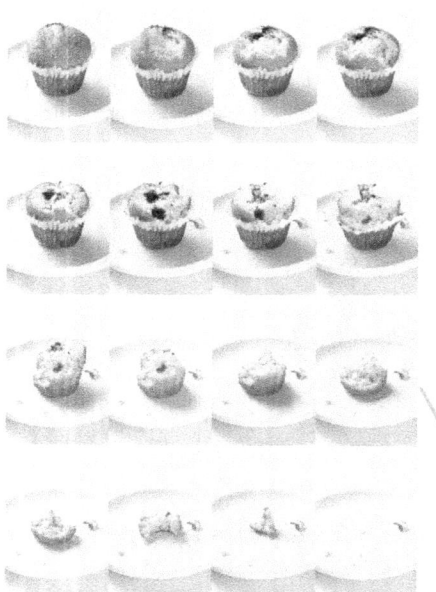

Note that I am not asking you to leave most of your food (Muffin) as in the top two rows. Actually you will do well if you can leave behind the amount of Muffin comparable to one of the squares in this row.

Remember, to apply the 20% Off method you need to avoid scenes similar to the picture below.

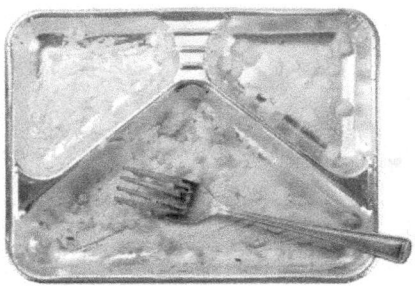

In the following examples, I will show pictures of how to apply the 20% Off method to different types of food and different situations. In all the examples, you need to follow the steps presented in the first example.

Example 2: Applying the 20% Off to a Home-Cooked Meal

This is an example of applying the program to a home-cooked pasta meal.

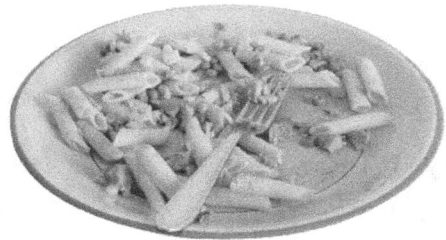

Example 3: Applying the 20% Off to drinks

Drinks also contain calories (but not water which you can drink as much as you want without adding weight). If you can decrease the amount of some of your drinks you will be able to reduce more calories of your daily intake which will contribute to more weight loss.

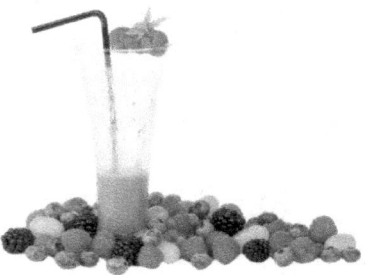

Example 4: Applying the 20% Off to a Pizza

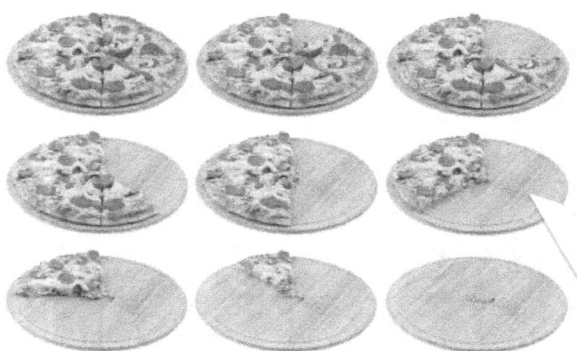

If you reach a point where you can leave half of your pizza, then you can switch to a smaller size. Doing so will save you money and will make applying the 20 % Off method more challenging.

Example 5: Applying the 20% Off at a Movie

This method will allow you to live a normal life and enjoy outside activities like going to see a movie. All you need to leave about one fifth of your popcorn or hot dog.

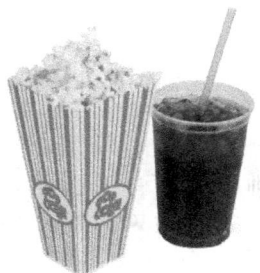

Example 6: Applying the 20% Off to a snack

For many people, over-Snaking might be the biggest contributors to their weight gain. The 20 % Off can be applied hear as well as shown in the pictures below.

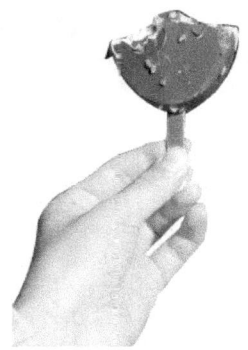
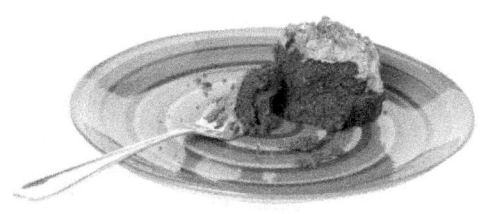

The picture below might seem little strange, but you can apply the 20% Off method to virtually any food you like to eat. However, if you like to eat a full box of chocolate (which is something I considered a hobby of mine) make it your goal to apply the 20% Off method to the extreme. By "extreme" I mean to work your way up on the amount of candies you leave behind to 80 or 90 %. This is because as you will see in part 2 of this book, candies are full with calories that are very easy to consume in short time.

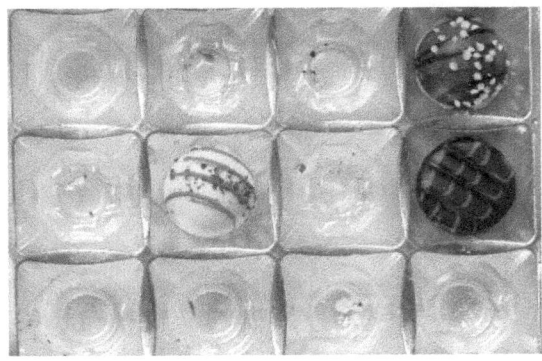

Example 7: Applying the 20% Off to salads and fruits

Actually, you don't need to apply the method on fruits and salads. However, you need to apply it on sauces and oils that you might like to add to your salads.

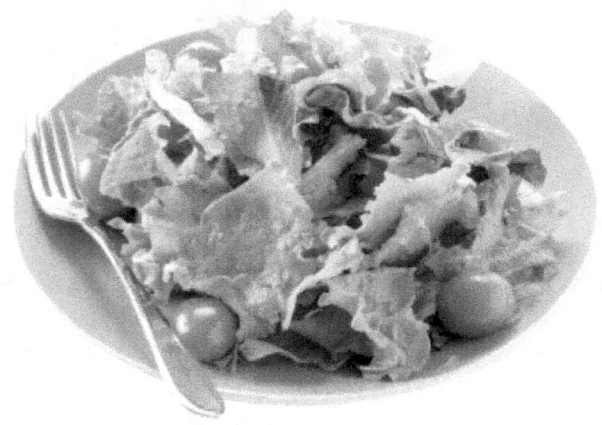

Fourth Element: Work on Re-Programming Your Mind

Great! Now you are taking pictures of your meals, so let's use them. You can use the pictures in the following ways:

1 As a proof that you are applying the 20% Off method.

2 You can analyze trends in your weight loss and make future plans. Pictures will not only capture how much food you left behind, but also the total amount of food you ate and from which food categories. This will help you understand how your body functions in relation to food and weight loss. For example, you might associate more weight loss with eating particular types of food. Also, you can trace back highs and lows in your energy level to the types of food you were eating.

For example, I had a period of 2 weeks when my weight was stuck and I wasn't able to reduce it at all. Upon checking the pictures I was taking with my phone, I noticed a trend, which was the introduction of iced coffee shakes to my diet in that period due to frequent visits to a bookstore that had a coffee shop. I experimented with eliminating that iced coffee, and I was back to making progress. To have a good analysis you need to do the following:

A Collect as many pictures as you can of everything you eat and drink.

B Take daily pictures of your weighing scale reading (note: as you will read later, I don't recommend using the scale for the first month of your diet, but then you should use it frequently thereafter).

C Dedicate a specific time in your day to reviewing the pictures of your eating and thinking of improvements. I prefer to do that before going to sleep.

After you have analyzed your data (i.e. pictures), you can plan for your eating by adding/removing foods as you see fit.

3 Reprogram your subconscious. Make it a habit to flip through your food pictures and think about them. Think about the quantity you ate and whether you are ready to decrease it. Think about the quantity of food you left and whether you can increase that. And think about the types of food you are eating and whether you can replace them with healthier foods. All in all, reviewing your food pictures, which proves your ability to control your eating, should reinforce your perceived strength over food, and your subconscious will be more inclined to make healthier food selections (either in type or quantity).

Reprogram your mind

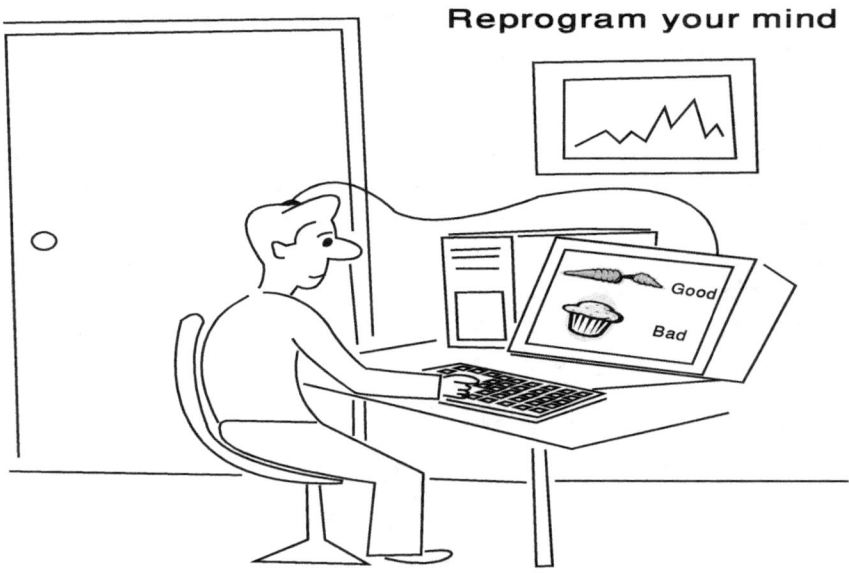

4 Feel happy about your progress. I remember when I had accumulated one week of food pictures, I was very delighted to see that I had adhered to the 20% Off method for the most part. This made me happy about my willpower, and it made me ready for another week.

To review your food pictures, you can just flip through them in your mobile or download them to your computer. I use both methods. I flip through them in my mobile when I am in a taxi or bus, before I go to sleep or when I am waiting to be served in a restaurant. I download them to my computer because I can arrange them by day and make a printout of them in that format (i.e. thumbnails of pictures arranged by day). After I print them out, I try to do some analysis on the amount of weight I have been losing and the types and quantity of food I have been consuming. It can be very fun; it's like I am becoming a food expert and teaching myself about the good and bad choices I made in that period of time, and it helps me make a plan for the coming days.

The following is an example of my food pictures downloaded to my computer. There are many applications that will arrange your pictures automatically for you.

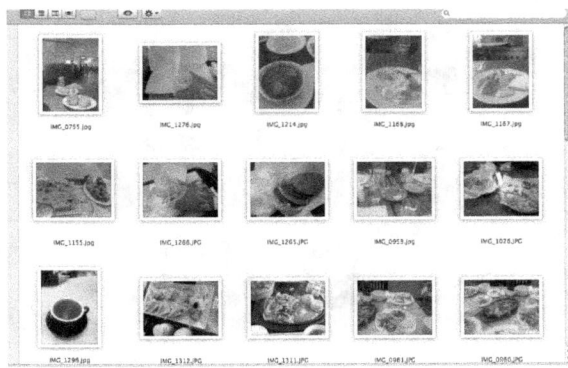

Getting Started Checklist

Now you have enough information to start on the 20% Off program. Keep reading through the book. You will see lots of useful information that will help you expedite your weight loss, but you need to start. This program is very practical, and you can use it not only to reduce your weight now but also to maintain a healthy weight throughout your life. Here is a checklist to help you start:

- Make an appointment with a doctor to check your general health condition.
- Make sure you have a mobile phone with a camera.
- Set a date to start, and tell your family and close friends.
- Take a picture of your current weighing scale reading.

Part II
Tools

In this part of the book, I will present some tools that will support your weight-loss efforts. This part is divided into the following four chapters:

- Know Your Environment and Plan Ahead

- Educate Yourself and Train Your Eyes

- Set Up Your Mind

- Invest in Yourself

Using These Tools Will Help You:

1 Expedite your weight loss when they are combined with the program

2 Continue the program until you start seeing some results, especially in the first few weeks

3 Adjust your eating program when you sometimes need to. For example, every now and then, you might not feel like you want to leave some food in your dish. During these downtimes, you may temporarily substitute the system with some of the tools and techniques presented here.

4 Steer, with minimal effort, the "elephant" of your desire to eat in order to walk on the path of weight loss. Read along to know more.

People who fail to stick to their diet are quite often accused of having weak willpower. An individual who is dieting might even be hard on him/herself, also believing this to be true. However, as laid down in the book Switch, by Dan and Chip Heath, the reason for failing at one's diet might not be that a person has weak willpower, but rather that he/she has used up a lot of that willpower to the point that there is no more to use in trying to diet. Like someone doing a bench press exercise, for example, the first reps will be easy and will gradually get harder, until the person is unable to lift the weights for anymore reps.

This concept in usually presented in psychological literature in the metaphor of an elephant and his rider. Imagine that your willpower is the rider, and that your desire and emotions are the elephant. Now, what if the rider and elephant had a disagreement? What if the elephant wanted to eat, while the rider wanted him to continue walking? Who do you think would win? I think I know who would win because I personally witnessed this dispute in 2003. I was on my honeymoon in Thailand, and I was riding an elephant with my wife as part of an elephant riding tour. Immediately after giving her passengers a ride, the elephant—her name was "Sugar"—seemed to stop quite often near some banana trees, but the driver used to steer her away. At first, he used to move her away from the trees by simply talking to her, and after a small hesitation she would continue walking. With time, however, he started to use his legs to press on her neck so that she would continue walking and he even hit her with a wooden stick. Ultimately, he used a metal hook on her head to steer her away from the banana trees (I asked the driver, and he told me that the metal hook didn't cause damage to the big animal). After about 10 minutes of this dispute, the Thai driver just gave up. He stopped trying to prevent "Sugar" from eating, and guess what happened? She ripped a whole banana tree from its roots with one pull with her trunk, a very powerful movement that made my wife and me afraid she would throw us from her back. "Sugar" ate for a couple of minutes, and then we safely completed our tour.

The lessoned to be learned from this story is that a small rider cannot prevent an elephant from having what she wants. Keep in mind that "Sugar" was a young female elephant, which the rider told us was very calm and easy to work with. What if the rider had had to deal with an older bull with big tusks? Now, I think you will agree with me that it would be unfair to accuse the Thai rider of being weak or not knowing how to manage an elephant. He tried, but in the end he couldn't withstand the might of the elephant. Similarly, your willpower shouldn't be blamed if it isn't able to stop the "elephant" of your desire to eat. Based on this story, you can also figure out why many people repeatedly fail in their weight-loss effort. They face a very powerful force telling them to eat, which is as big as an elephant, and they try to prevent it with the weak force of the rider. The above point boils down to a reality, that merely willpower is not enough to lose weight. You need tricks, tools and techniques that will motivate the elephant (i.e. your desire and emotions) to actually want to walk in the path of weight loss. These tools and techniques are presented throughout this book, in the elements of the 20% Off Program, and specifically in this part of the book. I have personally used all of them and believe they have had a profound impact on my weight-loss goals and that they should help you as well.

Chapter Four

Educate Yourself and Train Your Eyes

Read the Food Labels

For a long time, I heard about food labels and watched nutrition experts on TV urging people to read the information on these labels. Unfortunately, I thought that reading labels wasn't for me. I felt it would be "uncool" to check the nutrition information on every grocery item before I bought it. However, I was wrong, and have discovered that the information on these labels has a major effect on my weight loss.

If nothing else, food labels contain the single most important information about food, which is how many calories it contains. As mentioned in Chapter Two, calories are independent of the shape and weight of the food that contains them. This might cause you to wrongly judge the amount of energy contained in some food, and if you overeat food rich in calories, it will definitely contribute to your weight gain.

I don't want you to use a calculator to count calories that you consume. That will certainly be uncool. However, knowing the number of calories contained in the food you eat can help you achieve the following two goals:

1 Comparing similar food items with each other. As will be discussed shortly, you can reduce your calorie intake (which will later translate to a reduction in your weight) by choosing among very similar food items with varying amounts of calories.

2 Deciding whether the calories contained in a food justify eating it. To achieve that, you need to associate a meaning to the number of calories contained in each food item. For example, if I tell you that a cupcake has 500 calories, that number might not mean a lot to you. You need to benchmark such numbers to meaningful references. To do that, consider the following information:

A Average calorie requirements for men/women: To accurately determine your calorie needs will require a lot of calculations, but there are some starting points we can use. Calorie (energy) requirements are approximated to 2000 calories per day for women, and 2500 a day for men. So, if I now tell you that a cupcake will cost you 500 calories, and you are a female, that's almost a quarter of your gender-based normal daily calorie requirements. When you know this information, you can determine if it is worth spending a quarter of your daily calorie ration on a single cupcake. It might be worth it. I am not going to judge you here, but I want you to be conscious of your decisions. However, being conscious of the number of calories present in your food and comparing them with your total daily allowance of calories should help you to simply pass on many types of food that will consume large portions of your daily allowance. It's like having a daily dollar allowance. If you know that you have $15 to spend on food everyday, then chances are very low that you will exceed that allowance, and you will be looking for ways to save some of it.

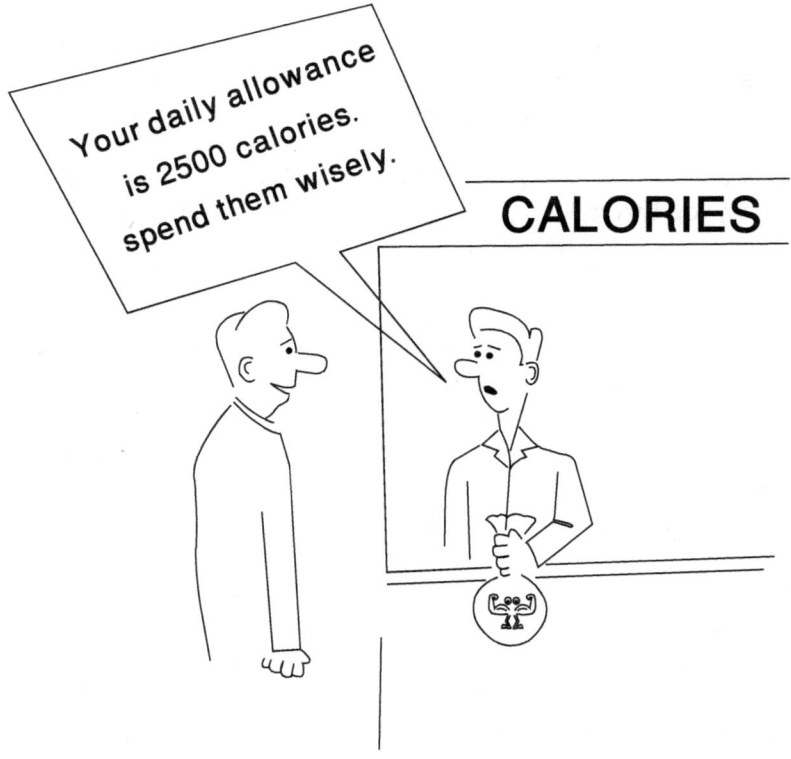

B   Set a benchmark for calories. Another way that will enable you to give meaning to calories is to know how many calories your favorite kinds of food contain. For example, my favorite food is a soft beef taco, and I like to eat three (3) of them in one meal. Now, I need to find out how many calories are in each of these tacos. This is very easy. Just search on the Internet, and you can find many available sites that will tell you the calorie count. In my case, I checked the website for the restaurant that makes the tacos and found that a single taco contains 190 calories, so if I multiply that by 3, it comes to 570 calories. Now this will be my benchmark—I know that for 570 calories I can eat the meal I like and be full and satisfied. I can now use the 570-calorie benchmark for other foods to judge their value to me. By value, I mean the satisfaction those foods will bring for the amount of calories they contain. So, going back to the 500-calorie cupcake example, I can justify to myself that it's very close to my calories benchmark, but it will yield me less satisfaction, so I will pass on it. I might say that a cupcake will occupy far less space in my stomach and will take less time to finish than the three tacos. This will cause me to feel hungry faster, so its value is small compared to the amount of calories it contains.

However, the matter of comparing food is not purely mathematical and doesn't depend on calorie count alone. It is rather complex and depends largely on one's feelings and mood. For instance, I might be willing to part with 20% of my daily calorie ration for a single cupcake just because I am feeling depressed, or maybe to treat myself for some achievement I have made.

I advise you to think of different favorite foods that you can use for benchmarking. In addition to your favorite meal, identify the calories in your favorite desserts, drinks and snacks.

Exercise: What is your daily calorie allowance? This information will depend on your age and weight, among other factors. Search on the Internet, and you will find free calculators that will identify this information with a great deal of accuracy. Search for the term "daily calorie needs."

Answer

Fill in the following table with your favorite foods to act as benchmarks for different food categories:

What is your:	Name	Calorie Count (You can use the Internet or buy books called "calorie counters.")
Favorite Meal (at home)		
Favorite Meal (outside)		
Favorite Dessert		
Favorite Drink		
Favorite Snack		
Favorite		

Using food labels in my diet was a real eye opener. I started to be more careful of what I ate and began comparing the value of different foods. People who don't know (or don't care to know) how to read food labels are comparable to someone who visits a foreign country and uses a credit card to pay for things without knowing the exchange rate between his currency and that of the country he is visiting. This will lead to many incorrect food selections. Please be careful here, since making poor food selections can come in two separate forms. The first is knowing that a certain food is not good for your diet, but you still eat it because you simply like it or feel you want it. The other form is that you don't know how a food item will affect your diet, but you still eat it without making any attempt to find out about it. The first form of poor food selection mentioned here is one that I can understand and actually empathize with; however, the second form is based purely on ignorance, and people who opt to do it will waste a great chance to improve their eating. To further illustrate my last point, I was amazed to discover that small changes in the food I consumed resulted in big savings of calories. For example, I didn't think of veggie burgers as good for dieting. I honestly thought they were introduced in the market to serve vegetarians' need for a replacement for meat. However, when I discovered that I could save 100 calories or more if I had a veggie burger instead of a meat burger, I immediately shifted toward consuming more veggie burgers.

The thing that annoyed me the most was that I didn't actually have any real preference for meat over veggie burgers. In fact, I liked veggie burgers more. In addition, a veggie burger was exactly the same size as a meat burger, so I felt as full. So there I was, due to my ignorance, adding many un-needed extra calories to my body without any real addition to my food satisfaction.

There are many foods that are similar in taste and size but that contain different calorie counts. Dr. Howard Shapiro, in his book Picture Perfect, gives many examples of such food, so you may want to check it out, or simply do a search of phrases on the Internet, like "options for food under 400 calories."

To use calorie information on food labels, you should do the following:

First, Appreciate and Accept Their Value:

As mentioned above, knowing about calories will help you avoid making poor food selections because you will be able to compare the energy (calorie) contents between different kinds of food. In addition, information about calories is well documented in scientific studies and widely available nowadays, and it's a fairly straightforward and easy concept to understand and apply, so I believe that failing to use them cannot be justified at all in the case of a person who claims to be serious about losing his/her excess weight.

Second, Know How to Read Food Labels:

Food labels are usually full of information like data on fats, carbohydrates and sodium contents. However, your goal is to find out how many calories (i.e. energy) are in the food. This is very easy, and should take you less than five seconds. All you need to do is to find the food label, and on top, you will see the calorie information. See the picture below for an example:

This refers to the number of calories

Nutritional Information	100ml	per serving of 15ml
Energy	2795 KJ 680 Kcal	419 KJ 102 Kcal
Protein	1.0 g	0.2 g
Carbohydrate of which sugars	0.6 g 0.6 g	0.1 g 0.1 g
Fat* of which saturates	74.5 g 8.6 g	11.0 g 1.3 g

However, sometimes you will need to convert a given figure of calories to understand it. Manufacturers often package food in containers larger than the amount that an individual can consume in one sitting. As a result, they suggest a number of servings per package. For example, you can buy a bag of candy that contains four bars of chocolate. But if you read the food label, you will find that the manufacturer is suggesting that two bars is the equivalent of one serving. This information can be found on food labels under headings like "number of servings per container," or " serving size." Let's analyze the information on the food label for a box of biscuits, as seen below:

NUTRITION INFORMATION		INFORMAÇÃO NUTRICIONAL	
Servings per package: Approx. 5		as porções por Embrulho: 5 Approx.	
Serving Size: 3 Biscuits (approx. 30 g)		que servindo tamanho: 3 Biscoitos (30 approx. g)	
	Quantity per serving* a quantidade por porção *	Quantity per 100 g* Quantidades por 100 g*	
Energy	612 kJ	2032 kJ	Valor Energético
Protein	1.3 g	4.4 g	Proteínas
Fat, total	6.6 g	21.8g	Gordura total
-saturated	3.6 g	11.9 g	saturada-
-trans fat	0 g **	0 g **	gordura de trans-
Carbohydrate, total	21.4 g	71 g	Hidratos de Carbono,total
-sugars	0 g	0 g	açucares-
-polyols	6.8 g	22.5 g	polyois -
Sodium	98 mg	324 mg	Sódio
**Not a significant source of Trans Fat *All values are average values		**Não uma fonte significativa de Gordura de Trans * Valores médios	

In the top left-hand corner, you will see that the manufacturer has divided the contents of the container into five separate servings, meaning that five people can eat the entire package in one go, or a single person could eat five separate servings. You will also discover that one serving size has been determined to be equal to three biscuits, which is equivalent to 30 grams. Now you will find different columns: one for the nutritional information for a serving size, and one for the nutritional content in 100 grams of biscuits. We are concerned with the first column on the left. The first entry in that column is for energy, which contains the number of calories in one serving size, which is comprised of three biscuits, which is 612 kJ. Hopefully, you noticed that the energy is given in kJ, which stands for kilo Joules and not calories. Kilo Joules (kJ) is just another unit for measuring energy in food, and one calorie has about 4.2 kJ. So all you need to do is to divide the number of kJ by 4.2 (or 4, for simplicity). Dividing 612 by 4.2 will yield 146, which is the number of calories contained in three biscuits.

So why should you be concerned about the number of servings? The obvious, and most important, reason is for you to avoid making mistakes, because for many people the serving size for many foods you eat in restaurants and buy in supermarkets is the whole container, whether it is a box of candies, a pizza or a can of soda. This can be misleading on many occasions when you will be happy to assume that some food will have a few calories, as stated in the food labels, only to discover that the calorie count is for just half of the food or even a lesser portion of it (based on the serving size stated).

Nevertheless, it shouldn't be difficult to work with food labels that show food divided into equal servings. For me, I almost always eat the whole container of the food in front of me, and thus I am concerned with the total amount of calories. So, I ignore the servings per container information (that is, unless the food container is very large). What I do is find the number of servings in the package and multiply it by the number of calories per serving. For example, if there are two servings in a bag of chips and 130 calories per serving, then the whole bag will have 2 * 130 = 260 calories. I will then use the 260 figure to compare the chips to other food options and determine whether I want to eat it and how much I should eat of it.

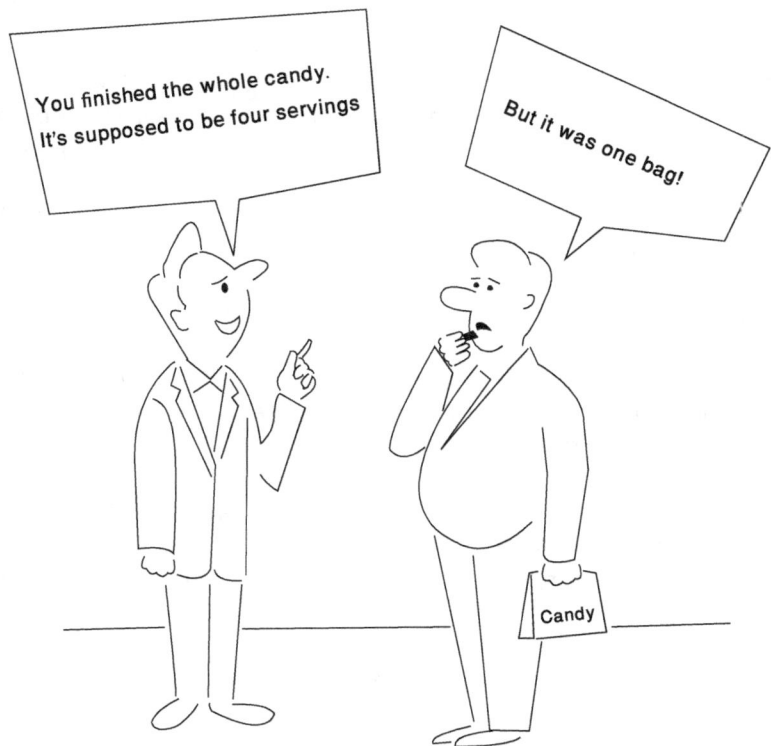

The first example for the box of biscuits contained an additional step of converting energy from kilo Joules into calories, but you shouldn't encounter this very often. This conversion is usually used only with some imported food products and, on many occasions, both calories and kJ will be stated on the food labels. Also, in the same example, the serving size was given in an easy-to-comprehend format, i.e. each serving was approximated to three biscuits. However, on other food labels, servings might be given in weight. For example, the food label might tell you that each serving is 30 grams. Therefore, to know how many servings are in that food container, you need to find the net weight of the food (net weight stands for the food weight, excluding the packaging). If the net weight is 150 grams, then dividing 150 by 30 will give you six—which is the number of servings in that particular container.

Steps in Reading Food Labels:

1 Flip the food container over to find the food label. Sometimes, the food label might be hidden underneath a flip top in the packaging, or be written in a different format (other than the table format) or a smaller font.

2 Determine whether the amount of calories given is for the whole food container or a portion of it.

3 Do any needed conversion between kJ and calories.

4 Decide to eat the food or look for an alternative— compare the amount of calories in the food and the potential satisfaction it will bring you both in terms of feeling happy and full.

Note No.1: Don't underestimate the need to read food labels carefully. Especially take note of the number of servings per container, as in many instances, manufacturers determine servings to be smaller than you might think.

Note No. 2: I have used the term calories throughout this book, but you will often find in literature and on food labels the term kilo calories (kcal)—they are basically the same thing, i.e. 1 kilo calorie = 1 calorie or (kcal = cal)

Note No. 3: Remember to convert from kJ into calories—you need to divide that figure (in kJ) by 4 to get the calorie value.

Note No. 4: Even drinks are often divided into equal servings by their manufacturer.

My Shopping Trip Report

Similar to a person traveling to another country and taking pictures of his/her sightings, I will present here my shopping trip with pictures I took with my mobile phone camera. I will show the discoveries I made, which helped me in selecting my food in a more effective way. After you go through this part, you will find an exercise to make your own shopping trip report.

On this trip, I tried to have an open mind. I imagined myself visiting the grocery store as a college student collecting information for a report on the calorie content in food. You can find much information about food nutritional content in many websites and books, but when you actually do this trip and touch and flip the packaging to find the food label, the information about calories will stick better in your mind, the same way it happened with me. In a sense, you will not be reading just to find information, but rather it will be like a journey of discovery.

Note: I want this section to resemble my actual shopping trip. For that reason I kept the pictures as they are (i.e. taken by an amateur photographer). You will notice that some food labels are difficult to read which is a problem I faced even before taking the shots

Variety: The first thing that caught my eye was the abundance in the variety of food items. There were many different brands of the same food item and, in many cases, they were not only different in price but also in calorie count. For example, in the case of candy, you might find ten different manufacturers, as seen in the picture below.

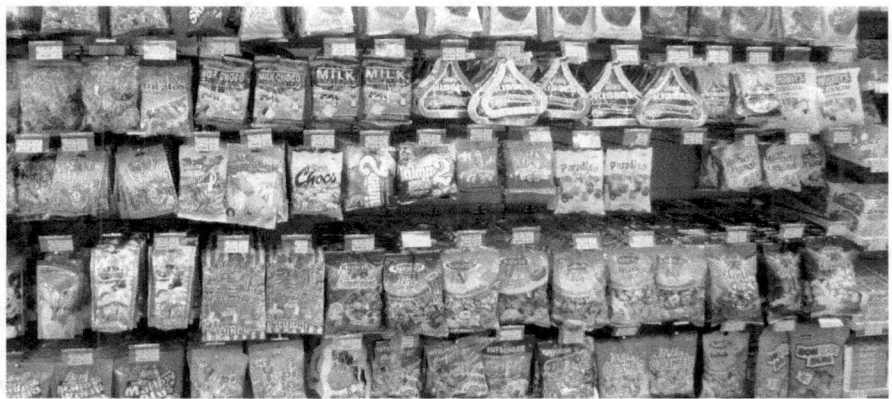

Calories in mayonnaise and ketchup

I found out that mayonnaise contains a large amount of calories in each tablespoon. I also discovered that there is "light" mayonnaise with fewer calories.

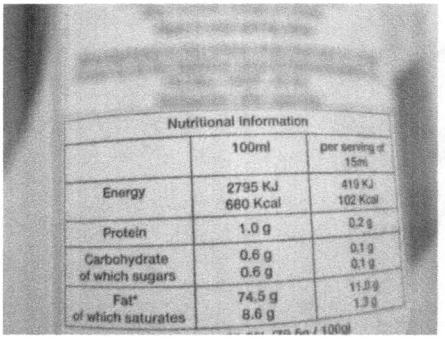
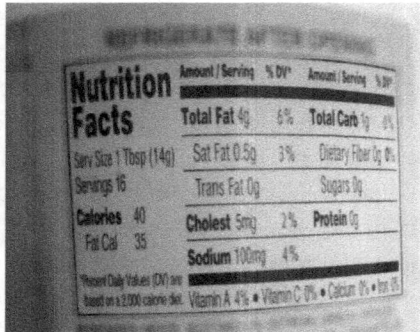

I discovered that ketchup has less calories, so I can still safely use it to add flavor to my food and feel comfortable that I am not consuming a large amount of calories the way I would with mayonnaise. As a matter of fact, the brand of ketchup I checked has less than half the calories of the "light" mayonnaise.

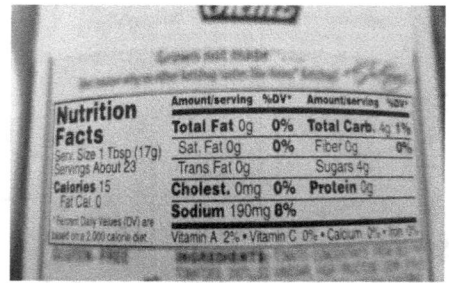

Calories in milk

I found that skim milk has a better calorie count than the full cream version (50 compared to 62). However, I was concerned that I would be getting less calcium with skim milk. After all, milk is known to provide calcium for healthy bones. An interesting thing I discovered was how the same manufacturer presents food labels differently. The amount of calcium in a full milk bottle was for each 300 milliliter (ml), and the one in the skim milk was for only 100 milliliter. So I had to adjust the amount of calcium in the skim milk by multiplying it by three (3), which came to exactly the same number as the one in full milk. So I opted for skim milk.

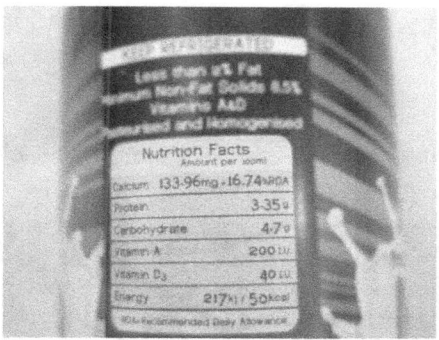
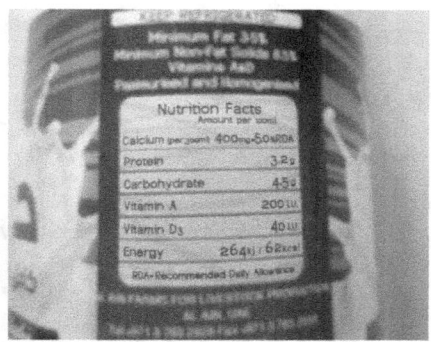

In addition, I compared chocolate and strawberry milk from the same company. The chocolate version had 90 calories, and the strawberry had 83 calories. This discovery not only increased my knowledge, but also caused me to realize that anything that contains chocolate will probably have more calories.

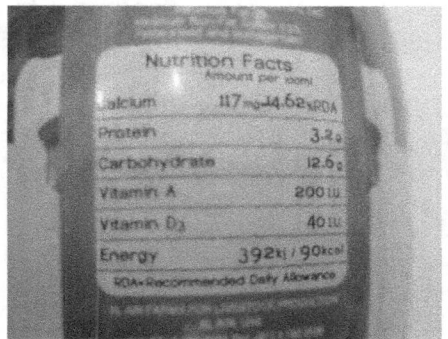
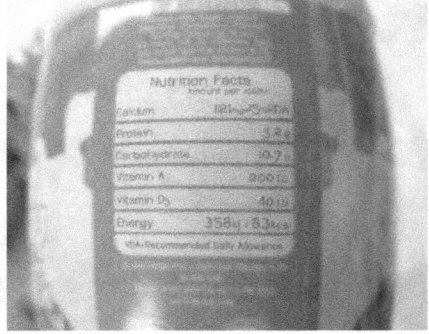

Calories in candy

In general, many candies have the same amount of calories based on similar weight, e.g. Snickers, Mars and Bounty bars. There are around 250 calories for every 50 grams of chocolate. This information can come in handy during instances when I cannot find a food label on some chocolates. Again, to put things in perspective, for 250 calories, you can eat a hotdog with ketchup. This last piece of information should help you compare between alternatives, and for someone wanting to lose weight, it's better for him/her to seek other kinds of food that are more filling. Think of the space in your stomach that a Snickers bar will occupy in comparison to that of a hotdog. If you choose the latter, you will feel fuller with the same amount of calorie intake.

Hint: Do a search on the Internet for "meals under 250 calories." You will be amazed at the variety you can find.

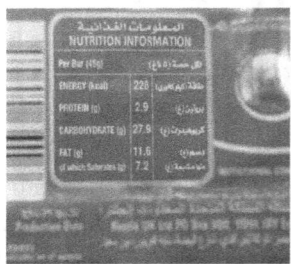 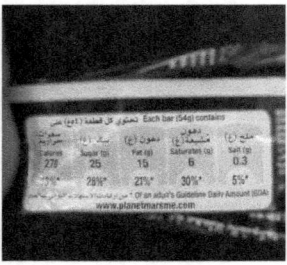 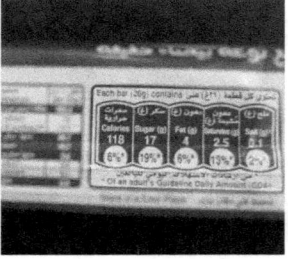

Notice that the calorie counts are comparable.

In the following picture, the candy package doesn't have a food label, but the calorie content is spelled out in paragraph form.

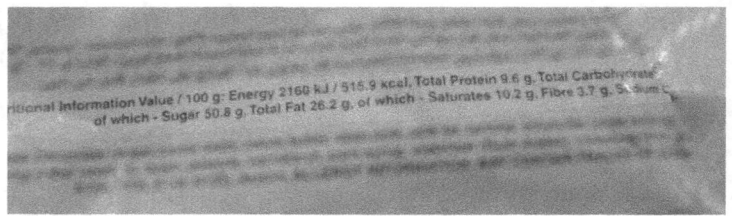

To illustrate how difficult it is sometimes to read a food label, consider the following candy, on which, even after zooming in with the camera, the writing is still barely discernible and is just too small to read.

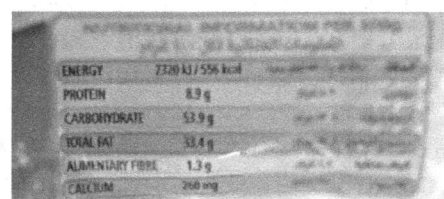

On the candy below, the food label was hidden beneath the packaging, so I had to flip it over.

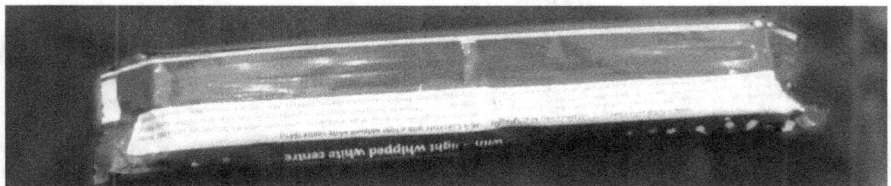

Calories in juice

The following piece of information was new to me. I actually didn't think that juice contains a lot of calories, or not alarmingly so, at least. I remember that during my college years, I met a friend late at night. He was walking around the campus and told me he was hungry and didn't know what to eat. Noticing that he needed to lose weight, I told him to buy a big bottle of juice and drink it all. "It will make you feel full and help you reduce your weight," I told him. "I think you should do this every night to lose weight," I added. Boy was I wrong! Just look at the pictures below, and you will find out that juice has plenty of calories. And the problem is, you will consume it fast, meaning that your pleasure in drinking it will end quickly, and you will be stuck with all the excess calories.

Personally, I tried to shift my drinking preferences more towards water. I particularly like flavored water with fruit infusions that have helped me in replacing juices. I also try to drink diet beverages as much as possible. Of course, I am not suggesting that you stop drinking juice (especially if it is fresh), but having less of it will help you reduce your weight.

I found that the serving sizes differ from one brand to another, like 100 ml or 200 ml. I also learned that milkshakes have more calories than other drinks, especially if they contain chocolate. Also, there are calories even in juices that claim to be 100% natural and "without any added sugar."

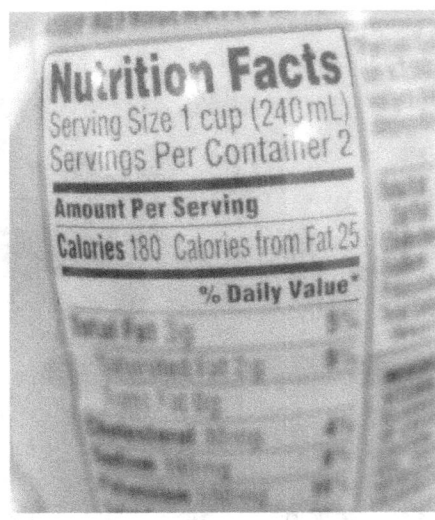

NUTRITIONAL INFORMATION L'information Alimentaire / Información Alimenticia / Informação Nutricional / المعلومات الغذائية النموذجية Serving size / Portion / Porción / Porção: 200ml / حجم الحصة الغذائية: 200 ملي لتر		
Amount per Serving / Quantité par portion / Cantidad por Porción / Quantidade por Porção / المقدار لكل وجبة		%DV / %VQ / %VD * % القيم اليومية
Energy / Énergétique / Energia / Energética / طاقة	100 kcal / 420 kJ	
Proteins / Protéines / Proteínas / Proteínas / بروتين	0 g	0%
Carbohydrates / Glucides / Carbohidratos / Carboidratos / كربوهيدرات	25 g	8%
Sugars / Sucres / Azúcares / Açúcares / سكريات	24 g	
Dietary fibre / Fibre Diététiques/ Fibra Alimentaria / Fibra Alimentar / إجمالي الألياف الغذائية	0 g	0%
Total fat / Lipides Totale / Grasa Total / Gorduras Totais / إجمالي الدهون	0 g	0%
Saturated fat / Lipides Saturés / Grasas Saturadas / Gorduras Saturadas / الدهون المشبعة	0 g	0%
Trans fat / Graisses Insaturées / Grasas Del Trans / Gorduras Trans / الأحماض فوق الدهنية	0 g	
Sodium / Sodium / Sodio / Sódio / صوديوم	5 mg	0%
Vitamin C / Vitamine C / Vitamina C / Vitamina C / فيتامين سي	25 mg	40%

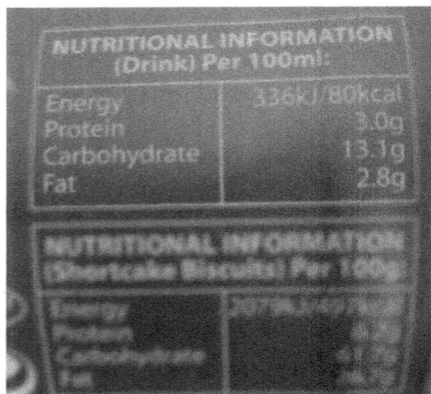

NUTRITIONAL INFORMATION (Drink) Per 100ml:	
Energy	336kJ/80kcal
Protein	3.0g
Carbohydrate	13.1g
Fat	2.8g

NUTRITIONAL INFORMATION (Shortcake Biscuits) Per 100g:	
Energy	

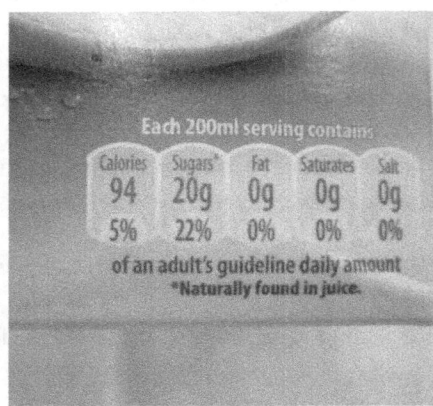

Each 200ml serving contains

Calories	Sugars*	Fat	Saturates	Salt
94	20g	0g	0g	0g
5%	22%	0%	0%	0%

of an adult's guideline daily amount
*Naturally found in juice.

As you can see, I benefited from my shopping trip and busted a notion that I have, which is juice doesn't have calories.

Calories in potato chips

I am not so much into eating potato chips, but my memory of potato chips comes from watching TV shows where obese people are filmed eating them. Indeed, on my shopping trip, I found this product to be full of calories, as per the pictures below.

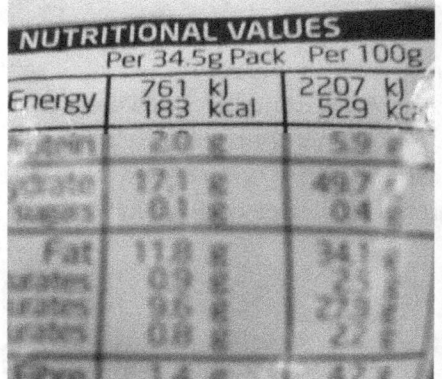

NUTRITIONAL VALUES	Per 34.5g Pack	Per 100g
Energy	761 kJ / 183 kcal	2207 kJ / 529 kcal
	7.0 g	5.9 g
	17.1 g	49.7 g
	0.1 g	0.4 g
Fat	11.8 g	34.1 g
	0.9 g	2.5 g
	9.6 g	27.9 g
	0.8 g	2.2 g
	1.4 g	4.2 g

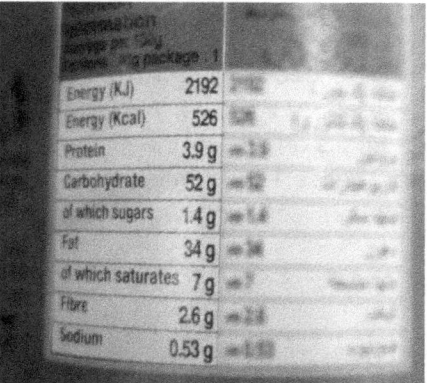

Energy (KJ)	2192	
Energy (Kcal)	526	
Protein	3.9 g	
Carbohydrate	52 g	
of which sugars	1.4 g	
Fat	34 g	
of which saturates	7 g	
Fibre	2.6 g	
Sodium	0.53 g	

However, I found a light variety of Pringles that claims to have half of the calories of the regular ones, so if I am ever going to have potato chips, I would definitely go for that one.

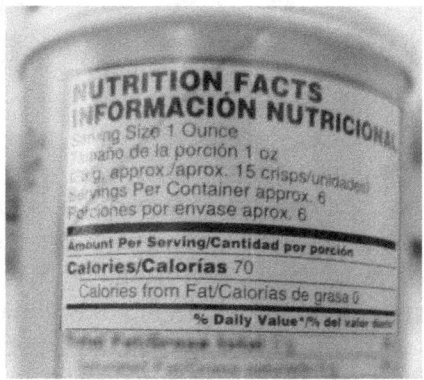

NUTRITION FACTS
INFORMACIÓN NUTRICIONAL
Serving Size 1 Ounce
Tamaño de la porción 1 oz
28 g, approx./aprox. 15 crisps/unidades
Servings Per Container approx. 6
Porciones por envase aprox. 6

Amount Per Serving/Cantidad por porción
Calories/Calorías 70
Calories from Fat/Calorías de grasa 0

% Daily Value*/% del valor diario

After taking the pictures of the two varieties of Pringles potato chips, I gave one package to my 4-year-old daughter and one to my 3-year-old son. When I went to check on them, I found that they both had finished their cans of chips regardless of the package size (my daughter got the small package with a net weight of 100 grams, and my son got the bigger package, which has about 170 grams). This didn't came as a surprise to me—we tend to eat all the food that a package contains, regardless of the manufacturer's recommendation of dividing it into appropriate servings.

Calories in cheese

I like cheese and believe it to be one of the contributors to my weight increase in the past. However, I found to my delight that there are low-fat cheeses on offer at the grocery store near my home. If I purchase the low-fat cheese, I can save several calories per slice up to half (60 calories for the normal slice, and 36 calories for a similar weight but a light version).

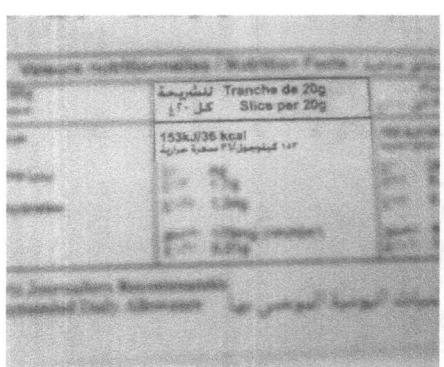 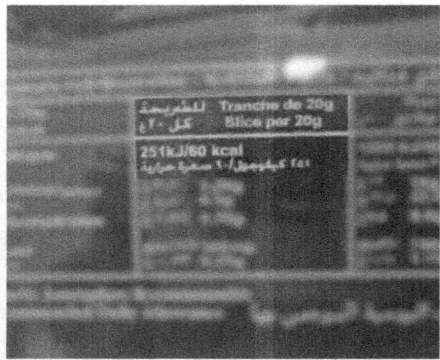

Calories in sweeteners

Sweets are major contributors to weight gain. Sweets are full of sugar, and many manufacturers have developed artificial replacements for sugar that don't have any calories but still deliver the same sweet taste, e.g. saccharin and aspartame. However, there is controversy on how they might affect one's health in the long run. People are divided between two extreme sides regarding these substances—as being perfectly safe or being carcinogenic (cancer causing). For me, I like to be safe, and try to avoid them as much as possible. However, during my shopping trip, I found a natural substitute for sugar (called Granola) that has the same calories but tastes four (4) times as sweet, so you only have to use a quarter of the usual amount. These natural sugar substitutes might not be very convenient (they are usually more expensive and not readily available in all stores), but they are worth investing in, especially at the beginning of your diet when you need every bit of help you can get to achieve faster results and increase the likelihood of your sticking to your diet.

COOK IT

Cooked desserts such as custard, milk and rice puddings can be sweetened with Sucron. Stewed fruit should be sweetened after cooking. Sucron is not suitable for jam making.

USAGE TABLE	
SUGAR	SUCRON
weight required in recipe	weight for equivalent sweetness
25g	7g
50g	13g
125g	32g
175g	44g
225g	56g
350g	88g
500g	125g

NUTRITION INFORMATION		
TYPICAL VALUES	PER SERVING 1/4 TEASPOON (1g)	PER 100g
ENERGY VALUE	15.8kJ/4kcal	1583.2kJ/371kcal
PROTEIN	0g	0g
CARBOHYDRATE	1g	98.95g
FAT	0g	0g

INGREDIENTS

Sugar, Sweetener (Sodium Saccharin)

Calories in bread

Bread might be the most difficult food item I have ever had to deal with diet-wise. This is because most of our diets have evolved around it. Even in earlier literature, you can find that bread was everybody's food: from kings to prisoners. The problem, in my opinion, is that our bodies grew to like bread so much to the point that, if we don't have it, we will lose our energy even if we keep consuming other kinds of food. One time, I tried the Atkins diet after it became an international bestseller. In a nutshell, all you need to do on the Atkins diet is to avoid bread (and carbohydrates, like pasta) and eat all the meat and cheese you want. I don't recall how much weight I managed to lose, but I have a vivid memory of how I craved bread. Bread was the only food item (other than water) that I couldn't resist, and for that reason, I had to quit the diet. I think that if prisoners were banned from eating bread and then punished by spreading the smell of freshly baked bread in their cells, it would be considered a cruel act of torture.

Going back to my shopping trip, I didn't manage to find food labels on bread in the grocery stores I went to. However, as a rule of thumb, each slice of bread will contain about 70-80 calories. It doesn't matter if the bread is white or made of wheat, both types of bread will still have very similar calorie counts. However, there is a real and documented advantage to eating wheat bread: it will take longer to digest. I did a difficult (and temporary) shift to wheat bread and found that I was able to lose weight faster when I ate it, and there is a simple explanation for that. Wheat bread has "impurities" (like the shell of the wheat grain). These impurities require more energy for our bodies to digest (than a very refined white bread), so more calories are burned—which is actually the goal of any person wanting to lose weight. As a matter of fact, you take more time chewing wheat bread to expend more calories.

It is well worth taking the advice to shift to wheat bread so you will lose weight faster. One problem, however, is that white bread tastes far better than wheat bread (usually because of the added milk and butter). It might be impossible to make a permanent shift from white bread to wheat, but at least try to have it as much as possible. For example, whenever, I go to a Subway restaurant, I try to order my sandwich on wheat bread. In addition, I try to have a variety of wheat bread that tastes better (but unfortunately costs more) like ten seeds whole bread. All in all, I have found that applying the 20% Off Program is the best solution to tackle my craving for bread. I get to enjoy the bread I love, but still have some control over my craving.

Calories in oils

Fats are the famous cause of heart disease and the most congested of calories among food items (9 calories per gram of oil or fat). I think we don't have trouble associating fat with weight gain because extra weight translates in our bodies as, well, fat. When I stopped at the oil section in the grocery store, I was looking to answer a question that has bothered me for a while: What about good oils, like olive oil? Do they have calories? Unfortunately, the answer is yes. It even has more calories than mayonnaise. So a food might be good and even healthy, but it can still increase your weight if you overconsume it. At this point, I want to emphasize the saying, "Decreasing the harmful is much better than increasing the good."

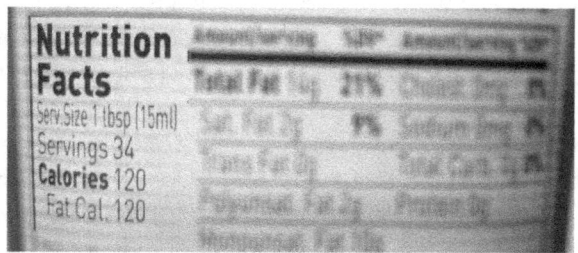

Needless to say, you need to reduce your intake of oils, oily food and food cooked in oil and butter, and I know that the 20% Off Program will help you achieve this objective with minimum frustration and hardship.

Note: During my shopping tour, I discovered the following new item, which is called "cooking spray." It basically has no calories and is used as a substitute to oil during cooking. My point here is not to urge you to buy a similar item, but to have a keen eye on new food items that may help you in your weight-loss efforts.

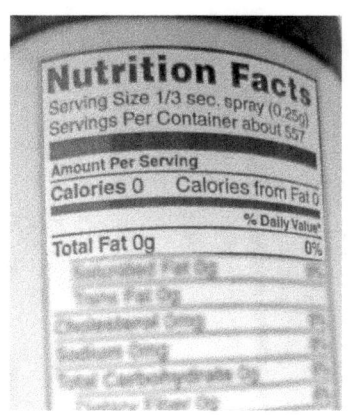

Exercise: Going on a Shopping Tour

Now I want you to discover the amount of calories available in the food you buy from your grocery store. You need to select a time when you are relaxed and the grocery store is not crowded. Walk between the aisles as if you were an inspector. Check the different food labels. Are they easy to find and read? Do they contain confusing information about the serving size per container? Can you compare different brands of the same food and find one with less calories but that has a similar taste and size?

This is an important exercise that I advise you to do. It will help increase your awareness about the food you buy. Just make sure you don't go to the store on an empty stomach, because "a hungry man cannot make good food choices."

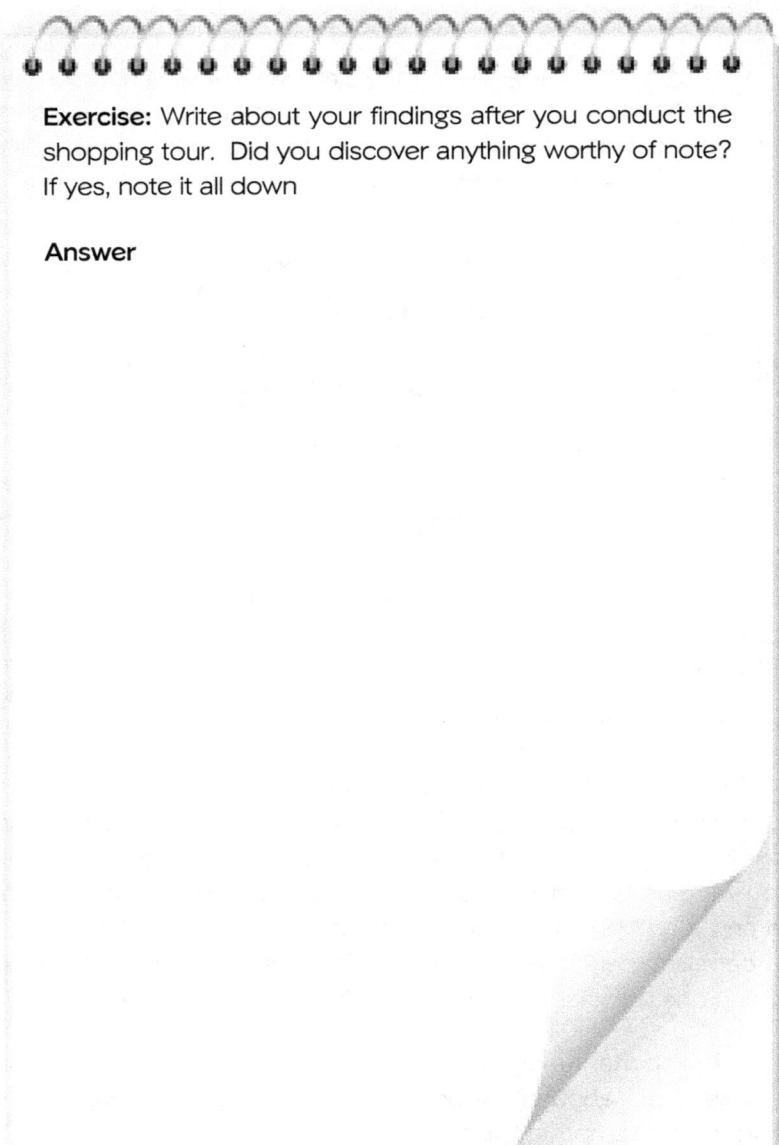

Exercise: Write about your findings after you conduct the shopping tour. Did you discover anything worthy of note? If yes, note it all down

Answer

What's Inside Food?

One day, I was surfing on YouTube and stumbled upon a video showing how to make mayonnaise. I was amazed at how it was made and didn't know that it contained the ingredients it does. After watching that video, I never asked for additional mayonnaise with my food and stopped using it as a dip for my French fries. But what about other foods that are rich in calories, like ice cream, milkshakes and cookies? Here, I will not include pictures of the different ingredients, but I want you to have the same experience I had. So search on YouTube for how these food items are made, and then you can decide if you need more of them or not.

Every now and then, I search on the Internet to find out how different food items are made, and always discover that large amounts of oil and sugar are used in processing different types of food. For example, I never thought that sugar is used in coleslaw salad, which is new information that led me to avoid that food. In particular, I advise you to search on how different sauces are made, because they are usually full of calories and, as I recommend in the next section, you need to consume less of them.

Lose the Extras

How important are the extras on your food? By extras, I mean such food items as mayonnaise, cheese and different sauces. For example, if I tell you that a Big Mac with cheese will cost you 576 calories, and a Big Mac with no cheese will cost you 495, will you be willing to leave the cheese out? For me, the answer is yes, and I will enjoy my Big Mac more because I will feel happy about saving more than 80 calories. How about if I tell you that you can save 50 calories if only you skim the mayonnaise away from the bun of your sandwich? I think you get my point, which is that small food additions (especially sauces) are rich in calories, and if you can avoid putting them on your food, then you can save a lot of calories.

What about salad dressing? Do you know that only two (2) tablespoons of Ranch dressing can contain up to 130 calories? Again, my advice is that if you can enjoy your salad without it, then you should do so. The list of savings in calories that you can achieve by avoiding the extras is very long. Many restaurants (and recipes for home cooking) advise the use of different sauces that are rich in oil and sugars. Personally, I think that using excess amounts of sauces and dressings is a trademark of sub-standard cooking. Anybody can make even a burned burger taste good if he/she covers it with a thick layer of cheese and mayonnaise. This is something I witnessed during my high school years, and I still remember it vividly. I used to buy a burger that tasted very good from a cafeteria near my house. I ordered so many burgers over the years that I struck up a friendship with the cook. One day, he allowed me to go into the kitchen to see how he made the burger. This is what he did after he put the meat patty on the bun: he put on a slice of cheese, then added a thick layer of mayonnaise and finally topped it off with a creamy slice of cheese. I guess nobody can go wrong with all those toppings, and I used to make jokes that if you replaced the meat patty with a piece of rubber, it would still taste good.

If you can manage to eliminate the extras in your food, you will save a lot of calories and can still enjoy the same food. However, if you cannot do that, then you can look for reduced-fat alternatives. For example, you can save up to 60% of calories by using light mayonnaise as against the regular kind.

Determine What You Really Want

One day, I was in a grocery store to buy a candy bar. I picked one up and was about to leave. Then I thought to myself: Do I really want this candy bar? Or do I just want chocolate, any chocolate? I realized I wanted any chocolate, and then started to consider the available options. There were many kinds with different calorie counts. The following are the pictures of what I considered to be my choices.

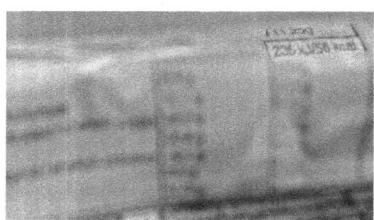
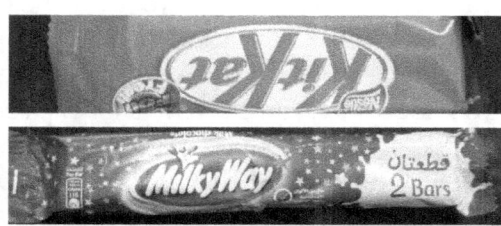

I ended up choosing a candy bar with only 56 calories compared to the first one, which had 270 calories. They were also comparable sizes. The first one had much less calories because it was made of halo biscuits and chocolate, and thus weighed much less. For me, it was hitting two birds with one stone. I still got my chocolate and saved many calories. I hope this example illustrates the benefits of reading food labels. In this instance, I saved more than 200 calories, which is a very good number of calories not to add to my body. As a summary, you can use this technique by following these steps: first, ask yourself about the food you want to eat. Do you want a certain brand, or doesn't it matter? If it is a certain brand you want, that's perfectly fine, and you shouldn't feel bad about it. But try to apply the 20% Off method on it. However, if you are indifferent to the brand, start considering the alternatives and select the one with the least number of calories.

Exercise:

Try to identify alternatives for foods you like that taste the same and have fewer calories.

Food You Like	Calories	Alternative Food	Calories

Learn to Say "No"

You need to educate yourself about marketing techniques used to sell you food you don't want or need. I believe it's fair for the food industry to look for ways to market their food, and it's your responsibility to choose among the food varieties available and decide on how much of it you need.

There is one marketing trick that I want you to be wary of, which can interfere greatly with your weight-loss efforts. It can come in many forms, but it is basically an offer for more of the same food with just a little added expense. If you saw the movie "Supersize Me," you will have an idea of how hard fast food restaurants try to make you "go big" or "supersize" your meal for just a few cents more. I had always fallen for this trick, and whenever I was asked if I wanted to have larger fries and a Coke, I agreed. I couldn't resist the good deal I was getting. For less than a dollar, I could get double the fries and a larger Coke. But this is exactly what the fast food chains (and psychologists, marketers and salespeople) are playing us with. It's the notion of a "good deal" that our minds are programmed to look for and accept. As if that isn't enough, you will be offered to "go big" by a nice and friendly person behind the counter … and our minds are programmed to usually just say "yes" to nice requests. But let me ask you, what if you visit a restaurant that doesn't offer a large size for your meal, are you going to ask for an additional beverage and extra French fries? I guess not, so we should fight against the urge to give in. Fast food restaurants care more about the one extra dollar they will get, and don't bother that much about the 300 or more added calories you will have in your diet. The solution is to say NO. This is not always easy. Saying "No" to other people might not be an easy thing for most of us, but with constant practice, you will master saying "No" when the occasion demands it. If fast food restaurants don't care about your weight, you should stand firm and say "No" to upsizing as much as you can. I recommend that you watch the film I mentioned above. It touches deeply on the subject of ordering more food (and the mentality that goes with it) and how it can affect you in an interesting and enjoyable manner).

Another form of this marketing technique is found in grocery stores, where you see signs like "Buy one & get one free," and food packages that say "20% more free." Of course, it would be foolish to not buy two food items for the price of one, but you need to be careful not to increase the amount of food you normally eat just because you are saving on cost. This is especially true with candies and sweets. So if you buy a Snickers bar with a 20% off tag, be careful not to eat it all. A nice trick is to cut the food items into smaller portions and store them in small containers and zip bags.

Low-Fat Food

During your grocery shopping tour, you will discover many food items labeled as "reduced fat" and "low in calories," or even "fat and sugar free." These items should help you in your weight-loss efforts. I particularly have skim milk, low-fat cheese and Diet Coke in my daily diet. Look for alternatives to the foods you like that are offered in lower-calorie versions. However, be wary of being tricked by the label of some food products that say "low calorie." Low calorie or fat free doesn't mean zero calories. One day, during a grocery shopping trip, I found a section for diet food. I purchased three or four candy bars labeled "fat free." I was happy that I could enjoy chocolate without guilt. However, I ended up eating all the candies in one day. Knowing that the food items were low in calories, I let down my guard and, as a result, buying the "fat free" candy bars caused me more damage than if I had eaten "normal" food. So, be careful that when you buy low-fat food, you make sure that you consume the SAME amount as you would if you were having the normal version of the same food. Otherwise, you will lose the benefit of that food and might actually end up consuming more calories.

In addition, in restaurants, you can ask the waitress if they have a low-fat version of the food you want. On many occasions, restaurants will be able to offer you low-fat sauces and cheeses. In coffee shops, you can also ask for low-fat milk.

The Weighing Scale

A good weighing scale is a must. It will provide you with information on your current weight status and how well you are progressing. I advise you to register your weight before you start the 20% Off Program (preferably by taking a picture of the scale reading). Then avoid using a weighing scale for the next 2-3 weeks. It's very important to avoid weighing yourself in the beginning of your diet. The reason is because you will lose weight very slowly, maybe just a few grams every day. So, if you weigh yourself after three days and find that you have lost only 200 grams, it is highly likely you will be disappointed and won't continue with the program. However, in due time, you will lose weight, and after 2-3 weeks on the program, your weight loss will be measurable and should give you a sense of happiness and achievement.

On the other hand, after the first 2-3 weeks, you should weigh yourself constantly, maybe every other day, so that you can track your progress and identify any tendency for you to gain some of the weight you have already lost. By that time, I don't believe a slow weight loss indicated on the weighing scale will give you a feeling of disappointment, since you will already have made some progress and won't be inclined to throw away the efforts you have made in the course of several weeks.

Create a New Baseline

In one study that investigated why inmates gain weight while in prison, the main reason was found to be due to their coveralls. Inmates in the study were issued loose overalls that hid their body, and this clothing made it difficult for them to spot the increase in their weight. Similarly, when you lose weight, your clothes will be loose on you, and you will enjoy the feeling of the extra space for a while. However, with the passage of time, this extra space in your clothes may encourage you (unconsciously) to slip back to becoming overweight again. Your loose clothes will prevent you from noticing (or caring) about one or two pounds of the weight you put on because it will not be visible. Be warned that gaining back a few pounds can open the door to more pounds until you reach your old weight and even go beyond.

Once you lose weight to the point that your clothes become too loose on your body, you should buy new clothes. This will help you set a new benchmark for further weight loss and help you see if you have started to relax in maintaining your weight-loss achievement.

When I lost weight, I went from being an extra large-sized guy (for t-shirts) to medium sized. However, I kept wearing my old clothes because they reminded me of my achievement and were cheaper than buying a whole closet of new t-shirts. But after a couple of months, extra weight started to slip back into my body and I didn't notice it immediately, nor did my friends point it out to me, since even they couldn't really tell my weight through my oversized clothes. By the time I started to notice that I had gained some weight back, I had already gained back about five pounds, and it was very difficult to lose them again. I believe it was more of a psychological factor that, when I added that amount of weight again, I felt worse because I had lost my guard. The idea of having to work harder to return to my ideal weight again that I had been at only a couple of weeks earlier was difficult to accept. To make a long story short, I managed to reduce my weight again, but it wasn't easy. Then I decided to buy a new set of clothes that weren't tight but that helped me to detect any weight gains in good time to make it easy for me to lose any extra pounds again.

Chapter Five

Know Your Environment & Plan Ahead

Planning ahead is crucial for your journey towards weight loss. If you stay at home all the time, you might be able to control what types of food you eat, and that might make it easier for you to lose weight. However, you definitely have to go out one way or another, whether it's for work, pleasure or to attend social events where you will be exposed to food that might not be the best for your weight-loss efforts.

You need to be prepared for such instances, because if you are prepared, you can enjoy your life outside and at the same time stick to your eating program.

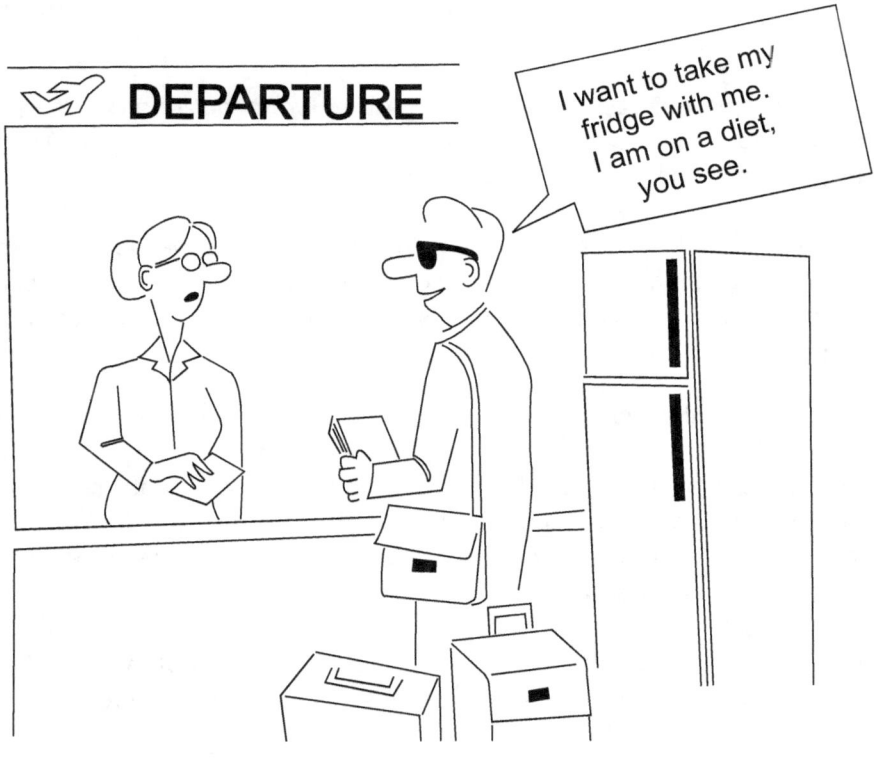

Where Do You Live?

If you want to lose weight in a relatively easy manner, you must teach yourself about your immediate environment and the available options therein. The reason is that there's a lot of good (and tasty) food out there with reasonable caloric content, but you need to know where to look for it. In my case, I like non-meat burgers that are made from vegetables or tofu. They contain less calories compared to their meat counterparts, and I don't feel there's much difference between them taste-wise. However, not many restaurants close to my home make them, and grocery stores have a very limited variety of them, if they have them at all. This has affected my food choices, since the food I like is not immediately available. I have had to make adjustments by selecting alternatives to my favorite food or planning ahead to buy the brand I prefer from distant grocery stores.

Some people may be fortunate enough to live in neighborhoods with restaurants dedicated to cooking healthy food with low calories. You may also live near one that you have never noticed before. To look for such places, you can always search on the Internet, or be vigilant about them and be on the lookout while walking in your town. As mentioned in the previous chapter, you should also go on "food discovery" trips to your local supermarkets and look for the types of food available, and match them with your personal preferences.

Another thing that you need to consider is whether you prefer to eat at home or out. If you like eating out, then make a mental list of the restaurants you should avoid (because they usually use too much oil in their food, or you are tempted by the variety of sweets and pastries they offer). It's far easier and, in my opinion, wiser to avoid such places that carry food that tempts you rather than going there and leaving it to your willpower to keep you from eating certain foods (the elephant again, remember?). Also make a list of the restaurants that serve food you like that will not tax your daily allowance of calories. You can make the list in the following exercise:

Exercise: List the restaurants that you should avoid to achieve your weight-loss goal. Note that you shouldn't boycott them, but it might be necessary to avoid them, at least when you start your dieting. If you don't know the calorie count in the food these restaurants offer, you may try searching online.

Answer

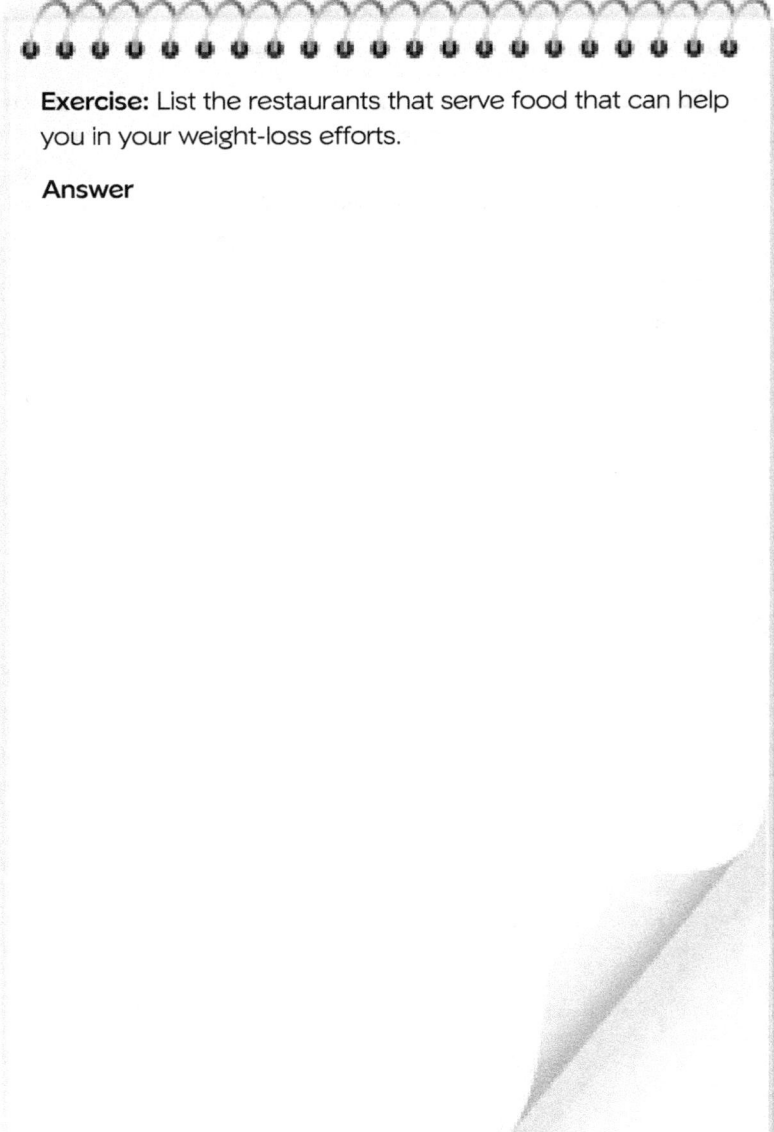

Exercise: List the restaurants that serve food that can help you in your weight-loss efforts.

Answer

What if you like to eat at home? Then you need to talk to the person doing most of the cooking (it might be yourself) and agree on recipes to avoid and recipes to introduce for a healthful diet. For example, if you live in a house with your kids and wife, who does most of the cooking, then you can negotiate with her to cook less fried food while you are at home. I used the word negotiate, because you need to consider her food preferences and that of your kids. Try to make a list of the foods she prepares in a week, and you will be able to identify dishes that she frequently or repeatedly cooks. From that list, isolate the dishes into food categories that are either good or bad for your weight-loss efforts. Then work with her and your kids, and encourage them to eat more of the good food on that table. This step should also include a review of your shopping cart to decrease the amount of foods not suitable for your weight-loss goals. For instance, you might ask your wife to buy less sweets, which will certainly not please your kids, but you can negotiate with them to at least decrease the number of sweets purchased or have them hidden from you. This will be discussed further in the next chapter under the topics "Win-win" and "What your eyes don't see will not hurt your heart".

Exercise: List the food you normally eat at home that are low in calories. If you don't know the calorie count, you can search on the Internet by typing, e.g. "calories in bread," etc.

Answer

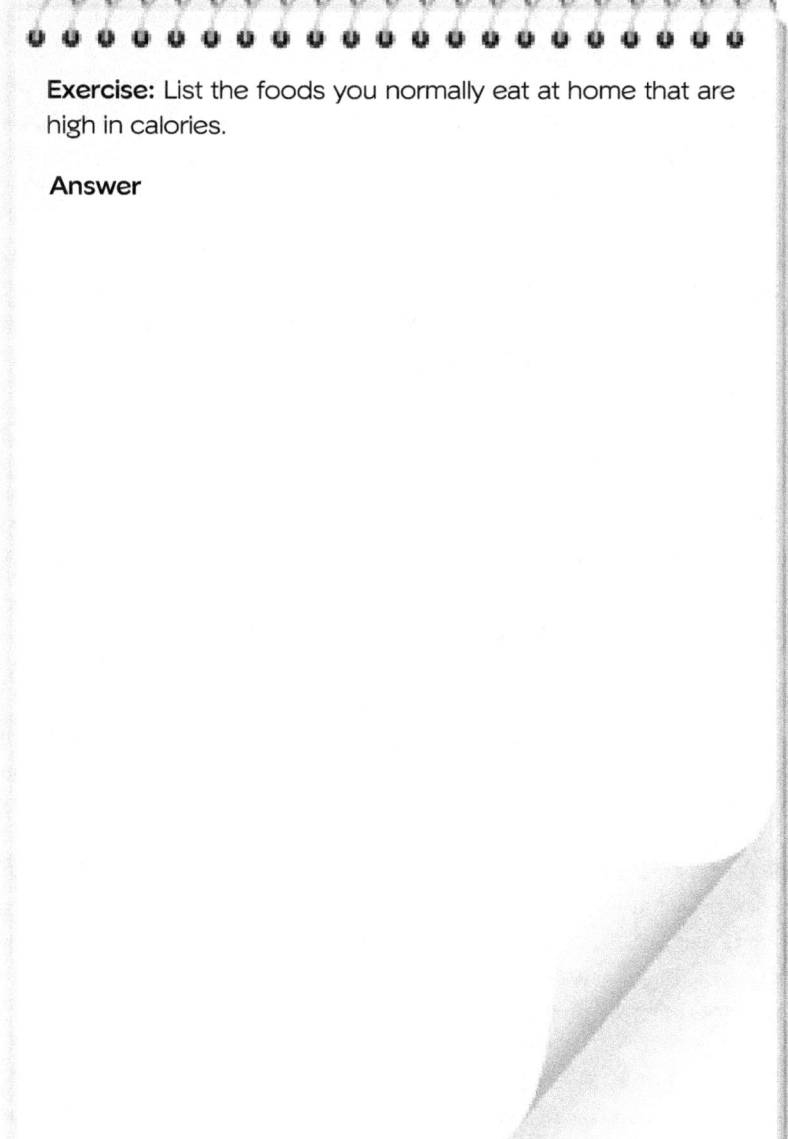

Exercise: List the foods you normally eat at home that are high in calories.

Answer

Eating Risk Management

This is by far my favorite tool and one of the most effective. It will help you avoid a notorious killer of balanced-eating programs, which is interruption. I've seen many people quit their diets because of a single interruption, and they go on to provide excuses like, "I ate a lot at yesterday's party, so what is the use of continuing?" This tool is very simple, and it guides you in planning your days in advance. It helps you anticipate any situation that might negatively affect your weight-loss program.

When you start expanding your knowledge base about food and nutrition, you will discover that there are many kinds of food that both taste good and are low in calories. Most likely, you will base your selections on your immediate environment, meaning you will look for different food options in the local restaurants and food shops close to your home or work. In time, you will get accustomed to these options and will be comfortable in selecting from among them.

But people today are very mobile. Even in a 30-minute drive, you can reach another city where you may not be able to find the veggie burger you like or that wheat bread full of fiber or that exquisite tofu hotdog. Add to that, when you travel, you are likely to be tired and hungry. And a tired man is not in a position to make sound food selections, especially in a new environment where he cannot find the food he is accustomed to. Aside from traveling to new locations, you will be invited to new restaurants and attend parties where you will be exposed to new food (usually in an exciting atmosphere).

This technique will help you avoid being vulnerable to such instances. It will not prevent the reasons why you might need to temporarily leave the environment that has the food options you worked hard to identify and enjoy, but rather it will help you live a normal social life without your having to break your new eating habits and quit your diet.

This tool is based on Risk Management, which has three basic principles: identifying, assessing and controlling risks. Let's explore them further.

Identifying Risks

Think about your upcoming day. Is it going to include any event that might interrupt your eating program? The best way of identifying such events will be based your experience. It might be that, in the past, you have always overeaten during a certain holiday, when going to a movie, on weekends or during vacations. These situations are specific to you, and you should not be ashamed to confess to yourself that you are weak in front of chocolate or a milkshake (in case you are). No judgment is going to be passed here. Just be systematic and logical in identifying risks.

Exercise: Can you identify situations where you are more likely to be prone to overeating? Also, list all types of food that make you lose control of your cravings.

Answer

Assessing the Risks

At this stage, you will determine how big a risk is. You should keep in mind two factors to determine the magnitude of the risk: first, the likelihood of it happening, and, second, the effect it will leave on you. We can represent this through the following formula:

Risk of spoiling your eating program = [**likelihood that** you will overeat] * [**severity** or calorie count of the food]

The elements of this formula are discussed below:

Risk of spoiling your eating program: This is the magnitude or score of the risk. It can be low, medium or high (or you can use numbers or different ways of scaling). The higher the risk is, the more effort you should spend to control the risky situation (which will be discussed later).

The likelihood that you will overeat: Here, you try to guess how hungry you will be in that situation and how much willpower you will have. You need to think about factors in an upcoming situation, like: your personal weaknesses (e.g. the weakness to resist the desire to eat a slice of apple pie), your energy level (whether you are tired or energetic) and the time that has lapsed since your last meal. You can give yourself a score of low, medium or high.

Severity: If you think that you will overeat in a particular situation or event, the question that follows is: By how much do you overeat and what type of food is your weakness? Are you going to add one more slice of pizza or an entire medium-sized pizza? Are you also going to drink a milkshake or a glass of orange juice? Basically, you are thinking about the amount of calories you will consume once you make a particular choice. You can also refer to this score as low, medium or high.

You might need help in computing the results of your risk score because you will have nine different possibilities generated from three possible results for both likelihood and severity (low, medium or high). You may use a risk matrix that looks like this:

Chance			
High	Medium	High	High
Medium	Medium	Medium	High
Low	Low	Medium	Medium
	Low	Medium	High
		Effect	

The small squares (9 of them) are what you want to be familiar with because they represent the risk score (i.e. the score that tells you how strict or relaxed you have to be when controlling a risk). To find which one of them represents the risk for your situation, draw a straight line from the likelihood and severity axis toward the inside of the matrix. The point of intersection will be the result you need. So, for example, in the situation of my being invited to a business meal in a coffee shop at 10 a.m., the likelihood that I will overeat is low because I would have already had breakfast, and I am not much of a morning eater (unfortunately, I am a big night eater). However, the coffee shop will most likely contain pastries and muffins, which I like a lot (and they are full of calories), so the severity is high. Now if I draw the two lines in the matrix, I will find that they intersect at a risk value of medium (as per the figure below).

Chance			
High	Medium	High	High
Medium	Medium	Medium	High
Low	Low	Medium	Medium
	Low	Medium	High
		Effect	

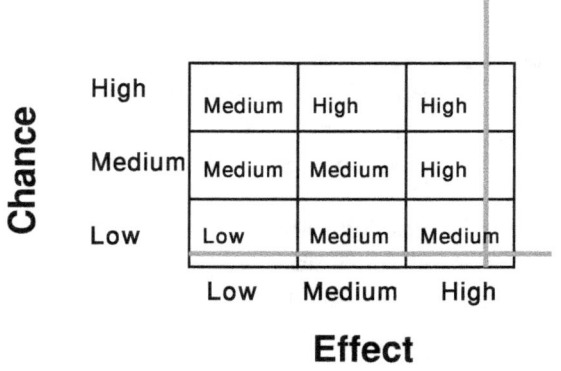

But what if I had a doctor's appointment at 1 p.m. for which I am required to fast 8 hours before? In that case, there will be no likelihood that I will overeat, and I run no risk of not following my eating program even if I go to the coffee shop (however, I then need to look at the situation after the doctor's visit and check the risk that I might overeat then, since I have been fasting for a long time).

This exercise of assessing the food risks on your program shouldn't take much time. Actually, you can do it in your subconscious without even realizing it. Consider another situation where you will go to see a movie one weekend. You might end up rating the chance of overeating as "high" because you reason that you haven't seen a movie for a long time, and you just can't watch a movie without snacks (it's your personal preference here, no judgment). You may also rate the severity as just "medium" because, although food in movie theaters is full of calories, they have also started to provide food options for people who are watching their weight. Therefore you may have just a "medium" likelihood and a "medium" severity, so that the risk will be "medium" overall, as per the risk matrix. Having a "medium" risk degree should make you think of a means to control the movie-going event, but without being too extreme about it, as will be discussed in the "Controlling risk" section.

Note No. 1: I want to emphasize that this exercise of assessing risks is very personal. Nobody will or should tell you that a certain situation will cause you to overeat or make bad food selections. You must determine that on your own, but it will require you to be honest with yourself. Use your past experience to aid you in identifying the likelihood and severity of risks.

Note No. 2: Don't be fanatic about the risk matrix. If you are not comfortable with it, you can just remember that the risk of spoiling your eating program will be low only if both the likelihood and severity are low. It will be high if one of them is high (or if both are high). For everything else, it will be medium. This is not a math book, but surely math is already deeply embedded in our life and will help you determine the magnitude of an eating risk. This should help you decide on how much attention you should devote to a particular risk.

Controlling the Risk

Here comes the most important part of the Risk Management technique, which is to think of ways to eliminate or decrease the risks to your diet. You can take one of the following three actions:

- Relaxed food control if the risk is low

- Moderate food control if the risk is medium

- Strong food control if the risk is high

In the "going to see a movie" example, the risk was medium, which, based on the above list of actions, will require a medium degree of control. Determining what is moderate control is highly subjective, and will be determined differently from one person to another. However, it would be helpful to think of what the two extremes might be and then select an option in the middle ground. In this example, the two extremes are either to skip going to the movie and stay at home or to have as much food as you want while watching the movie. Medium risk control may refer to taking steps that will enable you to enjoy your leisure time and maintain your eating program at the same time. An example would be to order plain popcorn and a Diet Coke. If you absolutely must have a hotdog, then discount the popcorn, or order the hotdog only with a little mustard and no mayo. The important thing here is to make up your mind NOW, before you are actually in front of the order counter with people waiting behind you. You are trying to avoid opportunities to stare at the food like a kid in a candy store. Remember, a hungry man cannot make sound food decisions.

I also found that merely thinking up a plan for what I will eat in a particular event makes the whole ordeal of standing in front of the food counter or party buffet much easier to deal with. I often picture myself in that situation and write down or imagine the food options available, and then circle the ones I should select. Believe me, it works like magic on the subconscious. Before we consider another example, let's summarize the actions you need to take to apply Risk Management to your eating:

1 Identify situations that might interrupt your continuing your eating program.

2 Assess the situation and decide how much it can impact your eating program.

3 Make a decision on what food selections you should make to reduce the impact of the situation on your diet. Make this decision now, when you have more control over possible sources of temptation.

4 Program your decision into your subconscious by thinking about, imagining and making a sketch of the situation.

5 Act.

Example

John just came from a meeting where he was tasked to travel from City A to City B and attend a business meeting. City B is only a 45-minute flight away, so his company booked him a return ticket on the same day. His flight is at 10 a.m., his meeting at 1 p.m. and the return flight at 6 p.m. The airport is a 15-minute drive from his home.

John is on the 20% Off program, so he starts thinking about his coming travel day using the risk management method.

Step 1: John identifies the travel day as an interruption to his program, because it will be a busy day, and he will have to be away from the environment where he has built a healthy network of food sources.

Step 2: John thinks that the chance of overeating is high, as well as severe because he anticipates that he will be tired from travel and will naturally go for fatty food to replenish his energy.

Step 3: To control his risk of overeating, he makes the following sketch representing a timeline and the available food options at each stage of his day.

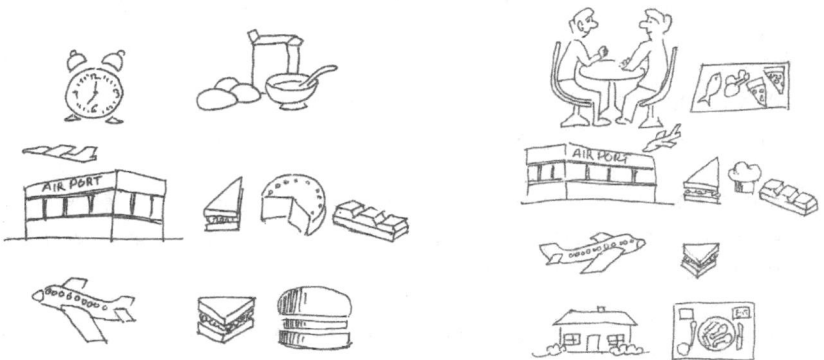

Step 4: John studies the sketch and comes up with the following eating plan for that day.

Time/Event	Food	Comments
Wake up	omelet + coffee	-
At the airport	turkey sandwich + orange juice	To have energy for the meeting
On the plane	-	-
During the meeting	coffee	Avoid ordering sweets
After meeting	Light lunch at the airport – tuna sandwich	
Dinner	Thin-crust home-delivered pizza	Medium-size and apply the 20% Off program. I will be tired, and it will serve as a treat for me for controlling my eating during the day.

John knows that he might not be able to stick to the plan. After all, unplanned risks can occur, like flight delays, or he might just have a bad day with low willpower in front of food. Nevertheless, he is correct in thinking that having a plan is much better than being unprepared. There is also a chance that he can stick to part(s) of the plan if not to all of it.

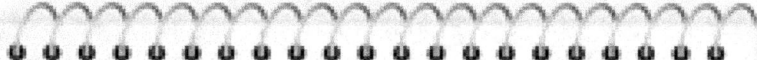

Exercise: Make a sketch of the food options that might be available for a situation like a meeting in a coffee shop (that was discussed earlier under the risk assessment section). Encircle the best options you have with justifications.

Answer

Rearrange Your Kitchen

Your kitchen is an important element of your environment. It can work for or against your weight-loss efforts. A sensible thing to do when starting an eating program is to have a close look at your kitchen and arrange it in a way that will help you in your quest to lose your excess weight. The most obvious thing you should focus on is the amount of food you have in your kitchen. If you are not afraid of an alien invasion suddenly happening, then you should store less food in your kitchen, thus decreasing the odds of eating more than what you need. In addition, you might want to remove candy jars from the kitchen (and other places in your house) and place candies in drawers instead, if you cannot avoid them totally.

After reading the book Mindless Eating by Brian Wansink, I discovered that the size of plates and containers affect the amount of food we eat and drink. The rule of thumb is, the bigger the container, the more we eat. As a result, I started rearranging my kitchen. I began with my spoons, and bought smaller ones. I also bought smaller plates for my meals and larger soup dishes (as soups will usually make me feel full faster and longer, and are mostly made of water, hence, they contain fewer calories). I also gave my big glasses away and bought thinner and taller ones that will hold less of a beverage but will give me a sense of "bigness."

You don't need to spend a fortune redoing your kitchen, but a closer look at what's inside your fridge and cupboards will help you identify some areas in which you can improve (they might be small steps, but an improvement nevertheless, like substituting the big spoons with smaller ones).

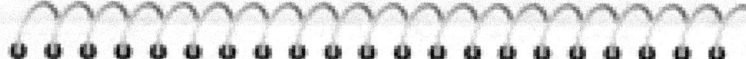

Exercise: Make a "person who wants to lose weight" inspection of your kitchen. Can you identify some improvements in line with the examples given above? If yes, can you execute them with minimal financial impact on you?

Answer

Avoid Excuses

The theme of this chapter is to prepare you to avoid making excuses. Risks to your diet cannot be prevented, but they surely can be reduced. Making plans regarding eating and arranging your internal environment to suit your dietary needs will help you avoid disappointments that can lead to your quitting your program. In addition, small preparations can save you from consuming more calories than you actually need. One weekend morning, I woke up to find a note from my wife telling me she had taken my son to the dentist and that I should make my own breakfast. I woke up late that day and was feeling quite hungry. I went to search in the kitchen and didn't find any food that suited me. I ended up putting 2 Snickers bars between two pieces of bread and making a Snickers sandwich. However, what if I had found low-fat cheese and skimmed milk in the fridge? If that had been the case, I would not have had an excuse to make myself a chocolate sandwich. I might still have had the chocolate sandwich (which I estimate contained about 600 calories), but at least I would feel less as a victim of not finding healthier food in my reach, and as a result, I might be more inclined to compensate for my actions by having a lighter lunch or dinner, or both.

In the first situation, however, I had excuses. Never mind if they were justified or not, they were clear in my mind. I was hungry on a weekend, when I believe I should enjoy a nice breakfast, and I didn't find any healthier food in front of me. The lesson that is to be learned from this story is to try to decrease the effect of chance having an impact on your everyday eating. Try to avoid situations that will give your subconscious excuses to overeat by anticipating them and preparing for them. As discussed earlier, using risk management and rearranging your kitchen is one of the best techniques to avoid excuses.

It is up to you to take full responsibility for your weight loss and to arrange your home to suit your purpose, so that you will be able to avoid situations similar to my Snickers story and save on consuming too many calories.

Chapter Six

Set Your Mind

Mind Setting

Simple thoughts and ideas can have a magical influence on us if they come at the right time and find a receptive ear. In sports, for example, coaches have developed many small mindsets to help their athletes perform better. I still remember when I was doing some back exercises at the gym in college, and was using my hands instead of my back muscles. The coach came over and told me to think of my hands as ropes attached to the weights. These simple words made a huge difference in my form, and since then, people have always complimented me on how I do my back exercises.

In this section, I will present simple words that carry deep meanings, which, if you embrace them and stay conscious of them, will have a profound impact on your weight-loss goals. You need to be conscious of these mindsets, but first, you need to be convinced about them. They represent what can be referred to as "common thoughts," but some of them might not appeal to you. However, there are many concepts discussed in this chapter, and I am sure you will find some that will be of interest to you.

The important thing about a mindset is how it can affect your eating and food selection. For that to happen, your mind needs to be aware of a mindset all the time. For example, consider the mindset that I will describe shortly after discussing "Something is Better than Nothing." Consider a situation where you are in a coffee shop, and the waiter asks you if you want your coffee with full or low-fat milk. In this scenario, you need to be conscious of this mindset even before the waiter asks you the question in order to enable your mind to make the following analysis: "The amount of milk in the coffee is small, so the calories I will save are minimal, maybe 10 or 20 calories, and this will not make a big difference to my diet. However, I accept that something is better than nothing, and saving 10 calories is better than not saving any."

In the beginning, when you embrace many of the weight-loss ideas described here, your mind might be slow in bringing them into perspective. For example, in the coffee shop, you might rethink the situation only after you have already decided to have full cream milk, or maybe you will not even think about it at all. The thing here is, you need to train yourself to think these thoughts actively and deliberately until they come naturally and effortlessly.

Something Is Better Than Nothing

I got this idea from one of my high school teachers. He always told us (students) not to leave any question blank in the exams. Even if we were not sure of the answer, we should try to guess and might just get the right answer. He reasoned that a mark of "1 out of 10 is better than 0 out of 10."

Before I embraced this mindset, I was often topping off damage to my diet with even more damage. But now I can at least stop at the first instance of damage, if it occurs. For example, when I overate at one meal, I felt that, since I had ruined my diet, I might as well go and have dessert even if I didn't want to. My reasoning was that I had messed up, and it would do me no good to control myself anymore. This is like saying that after eating a double cheeseburger that has 800 calories, it doesn't matter if I eat a candy bar that has only 150 calories. It will make no difference. I was telling myself, "Now that I've blown it, there is no benefit in continuing with dieting."

However, when I started to think that 1 out of 10 is better than zero out of 10, I was able to salvage those moments of weakness by refraining from eating even more food. Thus, I was able to save my body some extra calories. In addition, this sent a message to myself that there is no way out of my diet, even if I do badly at one meal.

There is a useful technique that can be employed by adopting this mindset, in which you will aim to achieve a reduction in your calorie intake no matter how small. I call it: "Play" with your food."

This is a technique that I use a lot, especially in restaurants. I eat quite often in these places and usually order the food as it is listed on the menu. For example, if a burger comes with sauce, cheese and pickles, I order it just like that. I know many restaurants will be happy to add/remove anything I want, but I like to order my food fast. I also speak so fast that oftentimes, the waitress asks me to repeat what I have just said. I have tried to overcome this habit. I have seen some waiters spend up to 5 minutes taking orders from customers, and they don't seem to be bothered. For me, however, I always give my order in less than a minute. Instead of trying to change my habits, I have tried to work around them (which is a mindset on its own—where you try to adjust to the words rather than adjust the words to you).

What do I do if I receive food items that I don't want and that will cost me some calories? I simply remove them. Like a gardener who trims trees, I remove the cheese and as much of the sauce as I can. For example, to remove cheese from a burger, I take a tissue and wipe the burger once to remove it. Whatever remains, I just ignore and eat it. I achieve two goals by doing this. First, I manage to work around my habit of not taking the time to specify what I want and don't want on my food. Second, I achieve some reduction in the calories my food would otherwise contain.

Another example is during travel. At the time of this writing, I was on an airplane and had just ordered a turkey sandwich. It came with thick slices of cheese, which I removed before enjoying my sandwich. I am happy to note that this happened at the time of writing this section. It supports my claim that the techniques used in this book are practical and can be used in a variety of places and situations.

To employ this technique, you need to have some self-control and remain observant of the food once it's delivered to your table. Don't just jump on it and eat it. Think of any reductions you can make in the calories of the food on the table. Even if the savings are small, taken altogether, they will count towards more weight loss.

Exercise: What do you think about this mindset? Do you agree with it? Can you apply it?

Answer

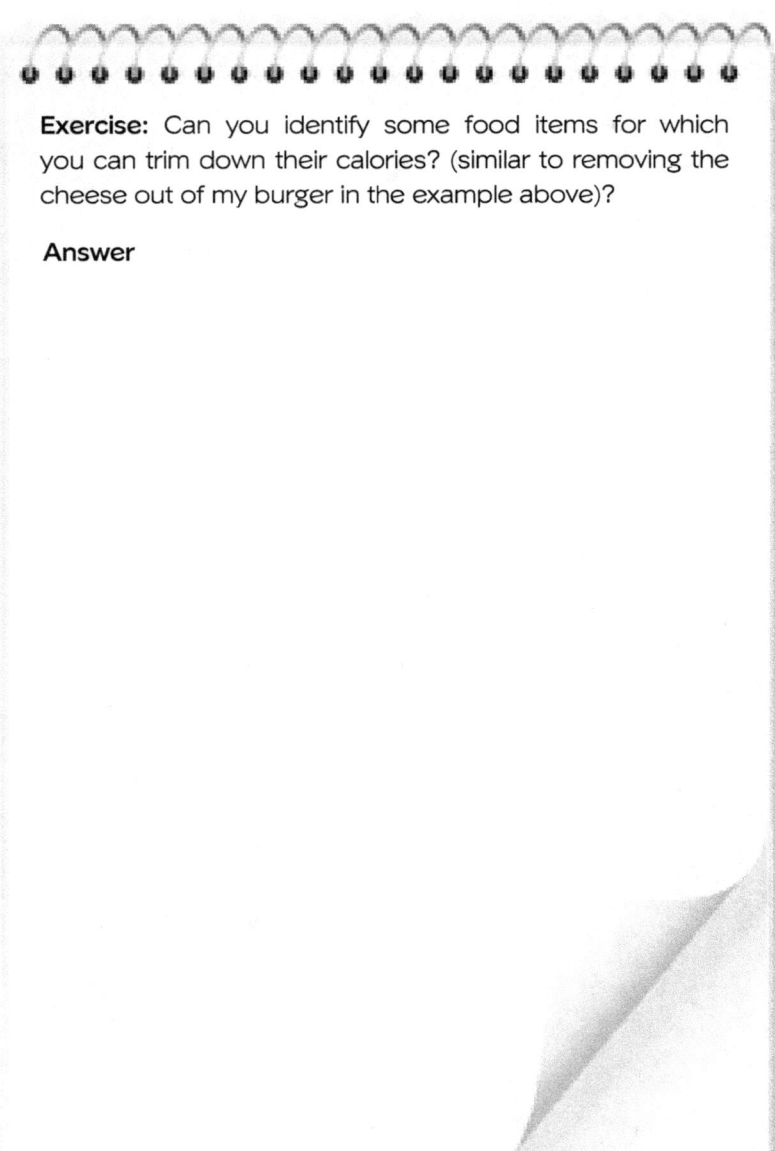

Exercise: Can you identify some food items for which you can trim down their calories? (similar to removing the cheese out of my burger in the example above)?

Answer

Look For the Positive Aspects in Failures

Earlier I mentioned the idea of a fat and a slim guy fighting to take control of our bodies. Based on this concept, when we are born, the slim guy is in control of our bodies, and for many people, the fat guy never wakes up. However, if the fat guy ever does wake up, it is almost impossible to put him back to sleep. This is a fact that I have accepted, to the point that, ever since the fat guy was woken up inside me, I now have a need to watch my eating for the rest of my life. I am similar to a person who is addicted to smoking—while he might be able to quit, the chance of his going back to smoking is still there.

All that it takes for the fat guy to be awakened again is one weak moment when you put your guard down. The aim of this mindset is to help you to never put your guard down. Even if you have spoiled your diet at one or two meals (or a full week), you shouldn't fall victim to the temptation of going back to uncontrolled eating. When I was writing these words, I felt bad about my eating one day recently. I started my day with a milkshake, and then ate candies and cake throughout the day. I also didn't apply the 20% system, and finished all the food that was in front of me, which wasn't a small amount. However, instead of just "losing it all," I thought of how I could compensate for that day. I actually used the "strong" feeling of guilt over my eating that day to make "strong" promises to myself to eat better the next day. Similar to a judo player who uses the strength of his opponent to actually defeat him, you can use the energy that emanates from your strong feelings to make strong commitments. By observing myself and others, I have found that when someone fails in a situation, he is actually able to make stronger commitments to improve when he realizes his mistake and consciously decides to mend his ways. The key is to capture the energy arising from the feeling of guilt and use it in the right way (i.e. towards the direction of weight loss). For example, you may have an issue with driving, say, and you may often be impatient with other drivers and always drive in a hurry. What if, in one instance, you drove fast and overtook a slow car and had a small accident? What if the driver of the other car were a nice old lady? Most likely, you would feel badly and make a promise to drive more slowly and behave yourself while behind the wheel. It's true that, in time, you might forget all about the accident and go back to reckless driving, but at least that feeling and the promise that followed made you a better driver for a while. Similarly, with food, you can have "accidents." The fat guy will wake up now and then, and will cause you to overeat or make bad food choices. Hopefully, you will feel badly about these instances, and then use those feelings to energize your commitment to better eating. As you can see, if you adopt this mindset, you can have many "accidents" in your diet as long as you make promises to recover AND you keep them. This mindset should help you to give yourself many chances to improve.

Let's take another example: Imagine that you came home late from work one night and found that one of your favorite movies was airing in half an hour. You saw this movie in college with your roommates while eating a Domino's Pizza. Naturally, the emotions evoked inside you on this night made you order a large pizza that you enjoyed along with the movie—you finished the whole thing! Even though you were aware that you were overeating, you continued anyway. To apply the right mindset, all you need to do is use the feelings of frustration in thinking of ways you can compensate for that behavior the next day. For instance, you can make a commitment to jog for an extra 15 minutes, or make yourself a low-fat dinner consisting of a turkey sandwich and a salad. Thinking of a "compensation" at the time you feel upset will most likely help you commit to that resolution. Note that I said you will feel "upset." I am not suggesting that you should go crazy if you mess up at times. On the contrary, you should take it easy, but strike a balance between your feelings and stay away from extremes. By extremes, I mean feeling miserable for overeating or feeling it's absolutely fine. You need a little reminder (i.e. the feeling of being upset) to prevent you from totally losing your commitment to your eating program.

Remember, we are working on the subconscious, which was programmed to make us eat the way we have for many years. Don't get upset, or worse, quit if you mess up with the 20% Off program at every meal of the day. There is always a tomorrow to start afresh with the program. The program will not quit on you. You can use it in any place and with any food. It's your life you are working on improving, so keep trying and be conscious of the good and bad food choices you might make.

Exercise: What do you think about this mindset? Do you agree with it?

Answer

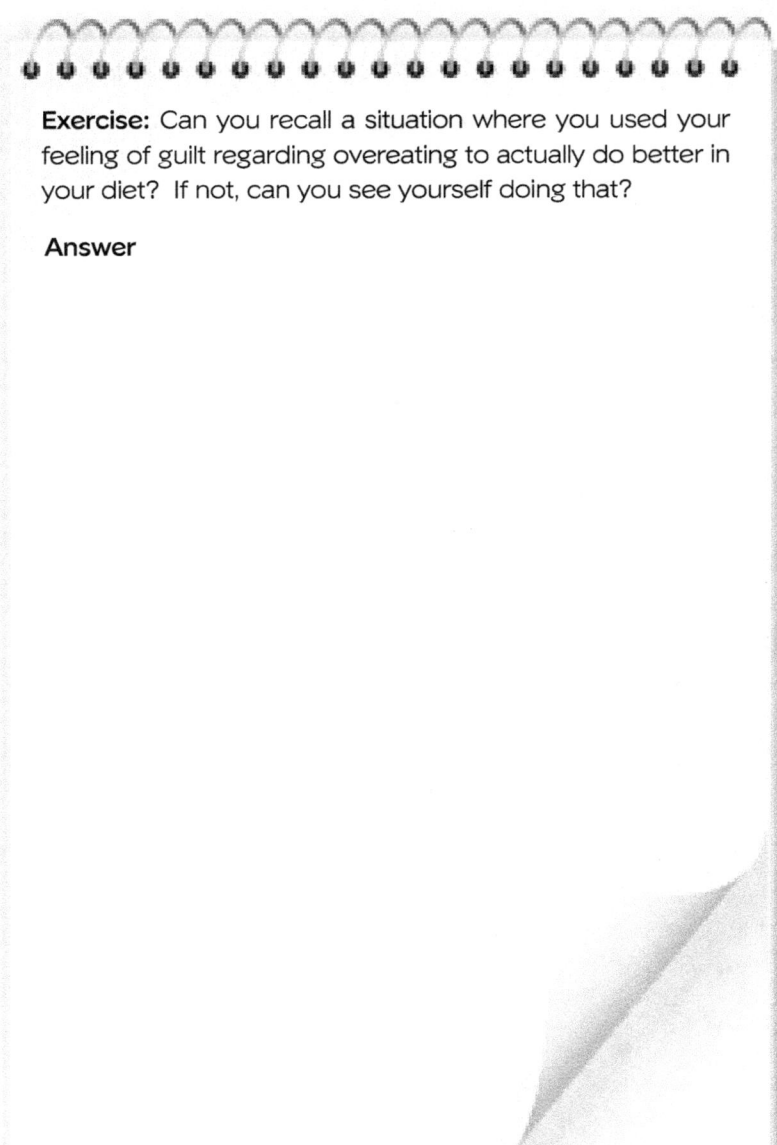

Exercise: Can you recall a situation where you used your feeling of guilt regarding overeating to actually do better in your diet? If not, can you see yourself doing that?

Answer

Exercise: Imagine that you were invited to dinner at your friend's house. Even though you controlled your eating for the main course, you absolutely blew it during dessert. You had two cups of ice cream and three slices of apple pie. What possible compensation for this situation can you plan for tomorrow?

Answer

Always Look For Win-Win Solutions

"Win-win" is a concept I always tried to use even before I knew it had a name. Its use is widely advised in management, especially during negotiations where every party in a conflict should get (win) something. Basically, it means to take what you want (or part of it), but give something in return. In your weight loss "life," there are two people: the slim guy and the fat guy. Both of them are part of you, and both have needs. The fat one wants to be satisfied with food (quantity and quality), while the slim one wants to feel in control of him/herself and make sound food choices. If you are overweight, no matter how hard you try, you cannot suppress one of them forever. What you can do is favor the slim guy and, in the instances when the fat guy wakes up, try to reason with him, give him something to eat and put him back to sleep fast.

Consider a situation where you are walking in a Sunday food market in your town. It's morning, and the weather is perfect. You see a food stall that sells waffles, and you start craving for some. You approach the stall and see that they have waffles with chocolate, which is your favorite syrup. To apply the win-win mindset, you need to talk to yourself and agree that a waffle with chocolate might not be the best breakfast for someone who wants to reduce her weight. However, if you prevent yourself from eating it, you will feel miserable. The best thing, then, is to take something and to give something in return. You can decide that you will allow yourself to have a waffle, but, in return, you will not choose chocolate as the topping, but rather have one tablespoon of honey.

In the previous situation, you managed to achieve two goals. First, you did not deprive yourself of the food you like. Second, you lessened the impact of the food (i.e. less calories) on your diet by "giving something in return." Actually you managed to achieve an even bigger goal, which is training to negotiate with yourself on the food choices you make. In essence, by applying the win-win method to your eating, you will be moving one level up in your dieting habits—to a level that involves less stress and fewer inner conflicts between your desire to eat and feel happy and your desire to feel in control of your eating. In addition, this mindset will teach you to balance and control your cravings, and it can be fun to apply, because you will use your mind in thinking about and balancing the different food options (i.e. balancing between the happiness that foods can bring and their calorie content).

Other examples of applying this tool are choosing to eat a burger and leaving the French fries in return, or having your burger and leaving the cheese out in return. Try to do the exercise below, and list as many situations as possible where you can eat the food you like by giving up something in return.

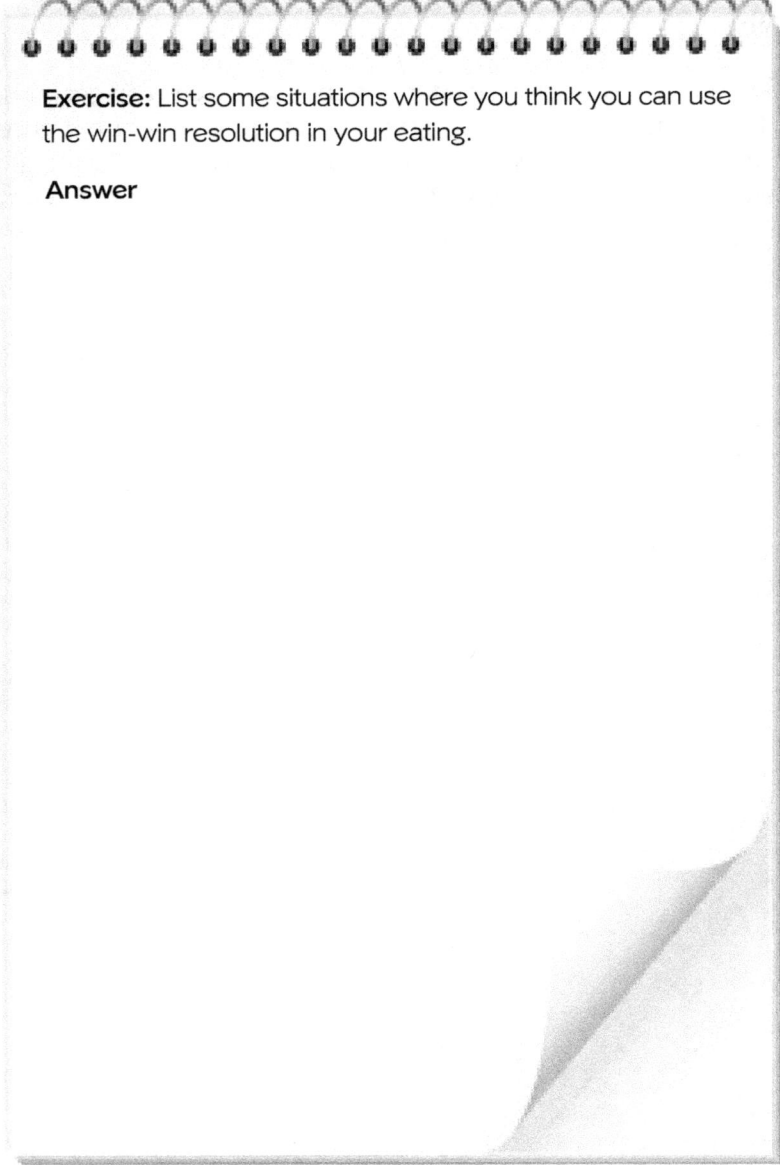

Exercise: List some situations where you think you can use the win-win resolution in your eating.

Answer

What Your Eyes Don't See Will Not Hurt Your Heart

Do you like psychology? If you do, then I invite you to try the following simple experiment. Fill up your fridge with candies and cake that you like. Then order a take-out dinner at home from one of your favorite restaurants. Don't order any drinks, as you will take them from your fridge. The next day, order the same take-out dinner from the same restaurant, but this time, order your drinks so you don't need to open your fridge at home.

Chances are that, on the first night, you were tempted to have some sweets from your fridge more than on the second night, simply because you saw all the sweets when you went to fetch your drinks. However, during the second night, when you didn't open your fridge to get drinks, the thought of having sweets was less likely to come to you.

I call on you, in this mindset, to try and avoid the sight of food that can make you fatter, like sweets and fatty foods. By avoiding the sight of such foods, you will probably think less about them, and hence, will not be constantly struggling with your willpower (and the elephant) to avoid eating them. However, unless you live in a cave, you will constantly be bombarded with advertisements all day long, and many of them are about food. Studies indicate that an average American can see between a couple of hundred and 3000 advertisement messages everyday. For that reason, you can guess why going to a wellness center on a remote island usually works— because you will be isolated from continuous and harmful food stimuli. However, there are some tricks that can help you avoid food stimuli in your environment, such as:

- Not filling up your fridge with sweets. Instead, try to buy your sweets on a day-to-day basis.

- Whenever possible, avoid walking near food stalls and restaurants. But don't be fanatic about it and start selecting routes that are long or dangerous just to avoid them.

- When walking near a restaurant or reading a magazine, try to control your eyes from focusing on the food advertisements.

- Ask people to be considerate of your weight-loss efforts. For example, if you are studying for an exam with your friends, ask them to not bring cakes and candies to the study room, or have them eat the sources of temptation before or after the study period.

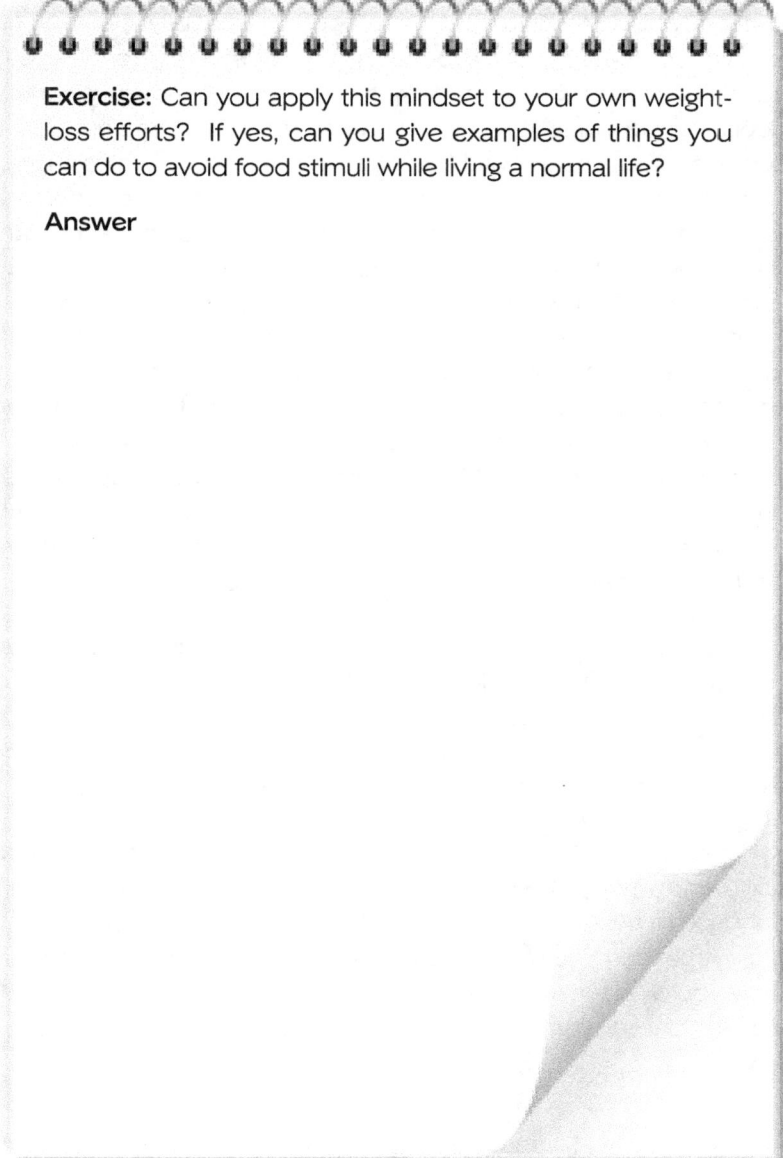

Exercise: Can you apply this mindset to your own weight-loss efforts? If yes, can you give examples of things you can do to avoid food stimuli while living a normal life?

Answer

Be Prepared to Feel Energized

One of the side effects of losing weight is having more energy. You might wonder how this can be a negative effect. Well, actually, it is not, but if you fail to harness the increase in your energy levels after you lose weight, it can actually backfire on you. Let me explain further: being overweight is usually associated with being less active and loving to relax (on your chair at the office or on your couch watching TV, eating your bag of chips). I know this stereotype is not necessarily true in all cases. As a matter of fact, when I was working in an oilfield, there were many engineers and technicians who were overweight but were nonetheless very active, since a lot of walking was required when working in an oil industry plant. However, for many people (including me), being overweight caused me to want to relax most of my day, especially when watching TV or surfing the Internet. Yet when I started to lose weight, I found that I had more energy than I usual. The thing is, when I was overweight, I arranged my daily activities based on the energy levels I thought were normal for my gender and age, but I discovered after losing weight that I had more energy. I had an excess of both mental and physical energy. I faced difficulties in sleeping, as my mind didn't want to shut down. I stayed focused longer and was able to walk faster.

The problem was, I wasn't prepared for all of that. I missed the nights when I would have a heavy late dinner and then would just sleep on the couch. But now, since such types of dinners were out of the question, I didn't know what to do with the energy I had. I was afraid that I would go back to overeating just to occupy the free time that was available to me.

In time, I learned to channel my energy to sports and found hobbies in reading and writing. I reckon that if I hadn't found hobbies, I would have gone back to overeating, because it was my only hobby for a long time. I call on you when you are in this mindset, to be prepared to use the extra energy you will have after losing weight. I advise you to look for a hobby or consider pursuing higher education and prepare yourself for a more active lifestyle.

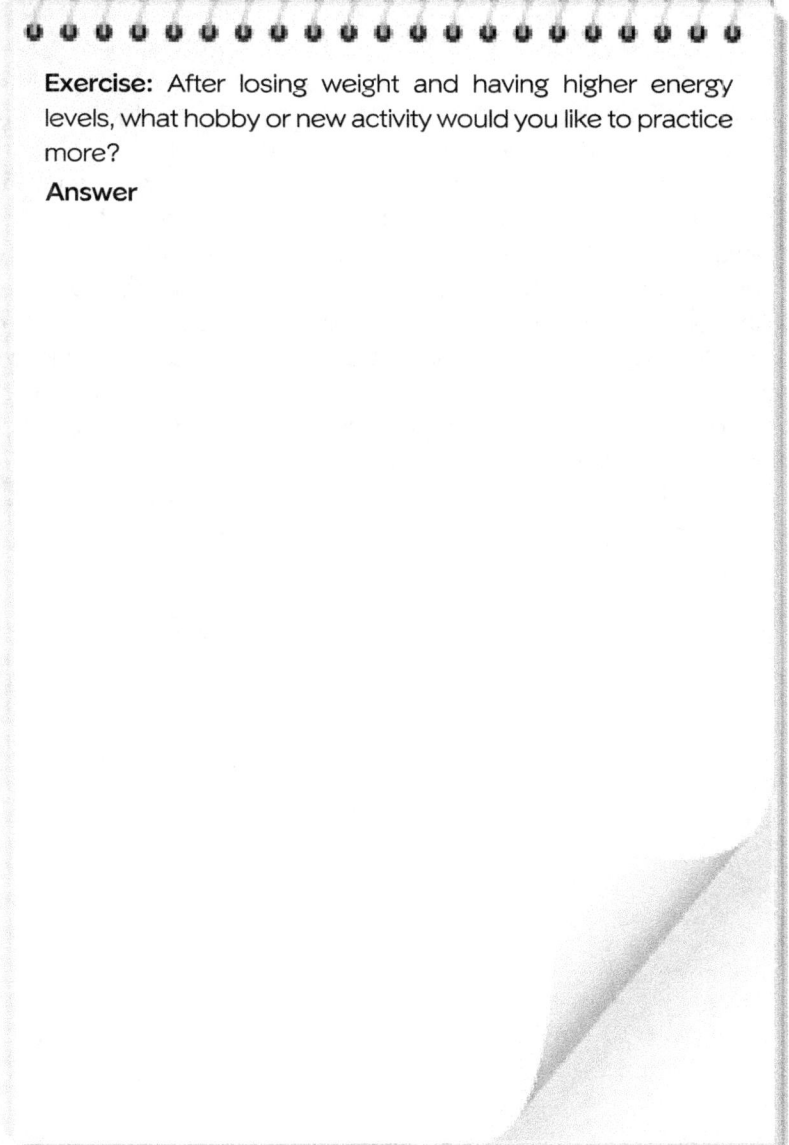

Exercise: After losing weight and having higher energy levels, what hobby or new activity would you like to practice more?

Answer

Don't Wake the Fat Guy Up

By the time you read this, it might be too late for you. As I mentioned before, if you get addicted to overeating, you probably will have to control your cravings for the rest of your life, similar to any other type of addiction. I call on you in this mindset to be a good deviant—to warn others from overindulgence when it comes to food, especially oily food and sweets. Now, after trying to lose weight, you know best that it's not an easy task, and you can talk about it from your own experience. You can warn your friends and co-workers, but more importantly, you can help your kids to not awaken the fat guy/gal inside them. You have control over your kids, so educate them about sound eating habits. Help them develop a taste for healthy food and practice a healthy lifestyle. I can't emphasize this matter enough, because at their very young age, you can teach your kids to eat right (and love doing that) so they don't feel deprived or unhappy when they avoid fatty food once they grow up. I feel envy for people who don't crave fatty food or sweets and still lead a happy life, while I always have to manage my eating. As a consolation, I can try to help my kids be in a better condition than I am.

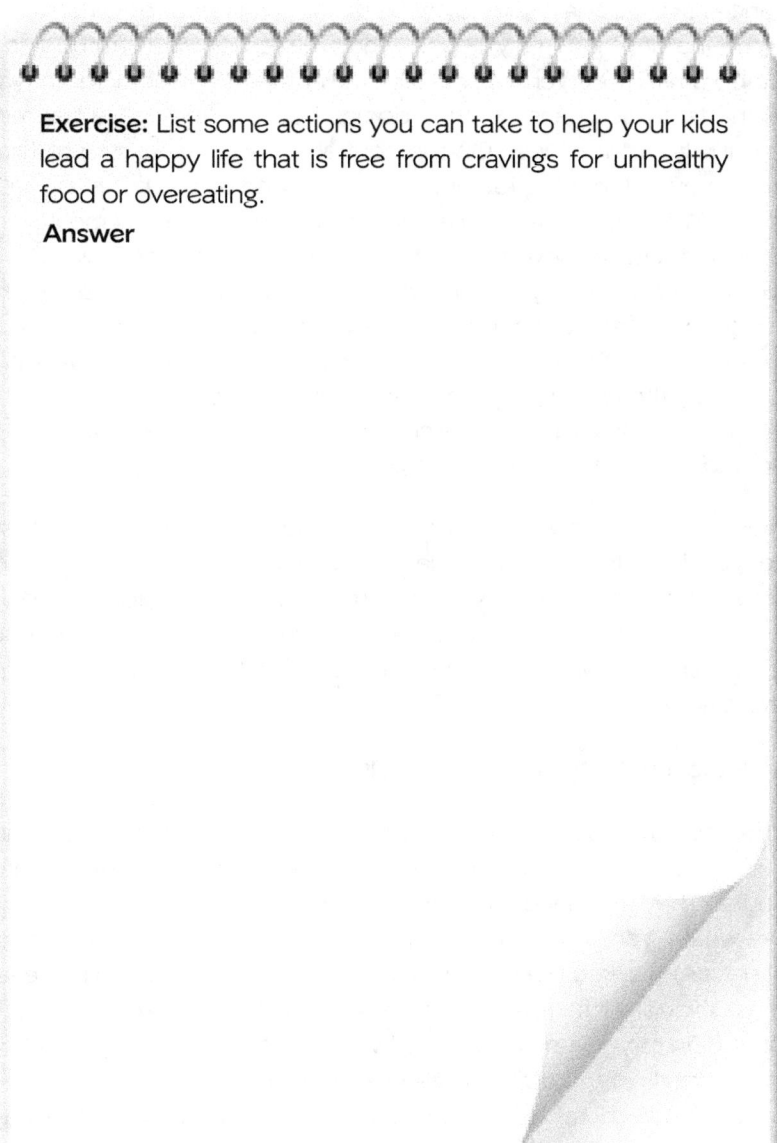

Exercise: List some actions you can take to help your kids lead a happy life that is free from cravings for unhealthy food or overeating.

Answer

Enjoy Your Weight Loss

Chances are, you have already realized that you need to work hard to lose weight—harder than many people who are blessed with slim bodies or fast metabolisms. However, you have an advantage over them, for they will not feel the fantastic change in their bodies because they have been slim for the entirety of their lives. On the contrary, if you manage to reduce your weight, you will feel the joy of a new body and all the benefits that come with it. When I managed to lose weight, I didn't spare any moment to feel happy about my achievements—from buying new clothes to walking up the stairs without losing my breath. In addition, I often compared my previous body to my current condition, which always filled me with joy. For example, I remember the first time I sat in an airplane seat after I lost weight. I was amazed by the extra space I had—not having 40 pounds to share the seat with me. Even small actions like crossing my legs gave me joy, since I wasn't able to do that in my previous weight condition.

In this mindset, always try to celebrate your achievements, because they give you incentives to continue in your weight-loss and weight-control efforts. They will also help you build memories of how good it feels not to be an overweight person and, in case you ever gain some weight back, the happy memories will help you lose the weight again, because you will know that it's all worth it.

Find Patience By Distracting Yourself

Life is fair. You didn't become overweight overnight, and you shouldn't expect to lose it in one day either. One time, I visited a weight-control spa in India. They had a weight-reduction system that required you to fast for three weeks from all food except what you could fit on a small plate (as your daily ration). I asked the doctor there how anybody could do it. He said, it's not as difficult as it seems. After the first three days, you will get accustomed to it. I didn't try this diet because I was staying for a short period of time, but the words of the doctor registered in my mind. It is the first three days that are the hardest, and if someone is patient enough and manages to get through those days, he/she will definitely be on a fast course to losing weight. But these three days (or any initial period in that regard) are the most difficult periods in any new program you start. The beginning is always difficult—it's like pushing a car that has stalled on the side of the road. First, you need to push really hard, but once the car starts to move, it will require less effort to keep it moving.

The concept regarding the first three days is present in all eating programs. You need to pass through a difficult initial period in your weight-loss efforts, and after that it should be easier. As a matter of fact, in the 20% Off Program, after the first couple of weeks, you will be amazed at how easy it is to control your eating and lose weight. However, you need to be prepared to pass the initial stage of the diet.

You need to look for patience and use it. This is easier said than done. But I found that it is a very useful technique to distract yourself. Find something you like to do and start it simultaneously with your eating program. An example could be starting an office improvement project at work that requires you to go back to the office and work extra hours. Try to choose a project that will take up most of your day so that you don't have time to think about food. It can also be a home improvement project, or one to convert your car to run on electricity instead of petrol … anything that requires all of your thinking and effort.

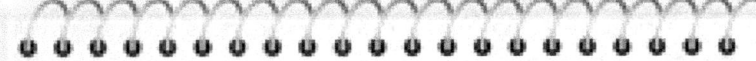

Exercise: Can you think of a project you can start simultaneously with your 20% Off program to distract you from eating?

Answer

The Conspiracy Theory—Fight Back

You will spend a lot of effort, money and emotions in reducing your weight. Nonetheless, there will be many people and organizations who will not care the least about that. Not that they don't like you or are all conspirators against your quest to lose weight. They just don't feel obliged to help, and will leave it totally up to you to help yourself. But who are those people and organizations? Well, take, for example, the fast food chains. Every year, they invent new food recipes that have ever-increasing calorie counts (how about a 1000-calorie burger—really, it does exist). Other examples are the marketing agencies that will collaborate with psychologists to present you with food ads that your mind cannot resist. What about your friends who will invite you to parties without making any arrangement for your special dietary needs? And people who call your diet a form of starvation? The list goes on and on.

In this mindset, you need to accept that the world is going in a direction that is the least supportive of people who want to control their weight. You need to fight back. Don't wait for help from the government to stop the selling of fatty foods or for your friends to serve only salads at parties. Take matters into your own hands. It's your life, after all. It is perfectly legal for fast food restaurants to train their sellers to ask you if you want to supersize your meal, just as it is perfectly legal for you to say "No."

I am not suggesting that you need to buy a camper and go live in the middle of nowhere. Learn to adjust to your environment and look for ways to fight back. This book is full of techniques that will help you fight back, but you should accept that it's your own responsibility to look after your eating habits.

It's Not a One-Time Competition, It's a Lifestyle

Many people manage to lose weight, only to maintain their achievement for a short period of time. A reason for this is that they view weight loss as a competition with themselves. They work hard to prove to themselves and others that they can do it, and many succeed in this. However, weight loss is not a one-time competition but a lifelong commitment. This last fact was the one that caused me the most worry. It is the long commitment that I was afraid of. I was scared of the thought that I would need to watch what I eat for the rest of my life. The idea of never again being able to eat a large pizza late at night was very hard to accept.

Nevertheless, deep inside of me, I knew that I needed to manage my weight for the rest of my life. When I accepted that fact, only then did I start to see results. Accepting that fact played a vital role in bringing me a sense of peace. This mindset of weight loss being a long-term journey made me take things slowly. I was no longer concerned with seeing fast results or looking for unproven shortcuts to losing weight. Instead, I fully adopted the 20% Off program and was very happy to see small but consistent results. I hope you will also look for small but sustainable improvement in your weight, because this is one of the most important competitions in your life. In fact, it will be your life.

Don't Shock Yourself Back Into Weight Gain

In the 20% Off Eating program, you shocked yourself to jump-start your weight loss, but be careful, since it can also happen the other way round. This is particularly true after you achieve your desired weight loss and are then somewhat relaxed in your food management.

I advise you in this mindset to be always vigilant of your feelings and changes in mood. It can be a vacation or the death of loved one that might cause you to become bored with watching what you eat and to go back to overeating. You might be tricked into thinking that you have become immune to weight gain, especially after months of success in keeping the extra pounds away. However, the reality is, it takes time to add weight back on, so even though you might not notice an immediate weight gain after you abandon your guards against overeating, the gain can still happen.

Consider the following example: You have lost your extra weight and were successful in keeping the weight off for a full year. Last month, your husband surprised you with a vacation to Paris for the whole family as a gift for your anniversary. You enjoyed Paris and particularly loved its atmosphere of abundance and its variety of restaurants. You relaxed during your 2-week trip and didn't bother much about what you ate. However, once you came back home, you noticed that your clothes were starting to get a little bit tighter, and that you were unable to control yourself against binging on sweets like before.

To analyze the situation, we can say that the trip to Paris acted as a back-shock to bad old eating habits. Most likely, people who stay on a diet for a long time will miss their old eating habits and will slowly slip back to overeating or indulging in an uncontrolled consumption of sweets and other dangerous temptations. In this mindset, I advise you to accept that possibility (i.e. the possibility of going back to your old eating habits) and be prepared to work around it if it does happen. The first thing to do, of course, is to try to prevent such back-shocks from happening. If we consider the trip to Paris example, you could plan ahead for your trip by using the "food risk assessment" technique mentioned earlier. The second thing is to know exactly when you are slipping into a back-shock. You will notice a change in your commitment toward managing your food and a general boredom with your current eating habits. What I advise you to do in this stage is to take it easy and not to ignore your desire to make different eating selections. The fat man is trying to wake up and take full control of your body again; you don't want to fight with him because he was asleep for a long time and will have more incentives to be in control again, unlike the slim man, who is becoming more relaxed after achieving his goal of losing weight. What you can do is apply the win-win resolution and allow your body to release any tension it has accumulated during your long diet and to have the food it craves. However, slowly try to get back to the eating program. For example, you can allow yourself to eat more sweets but then you should exercise more as well. Try to introduce a variety to your lifestyle to avoid boredom, such as new food that is both tasty and easy on the calories. Even minor changes can make a difference, so always look for new things. For example, I visited a French café with my wife, and the waiters suggested that I try muesli, which is made of cereals combined with low-fat strawberry yogurt. Up until then, I thought I had tried every food that was low in calories and tasted good, but I really liked muesli, and it was a welcome addition to my "no guilt" food list.

It is important to understand that you can go back to being overweight, but don't let this idea haunt you to such a degree that you are in constant fear of it. All that you need to do is to watch your weight, and once you see signs that you are gaining weight again, you should have a time-out and think about why this is happening. Then take small but consistent steps to get back on track.

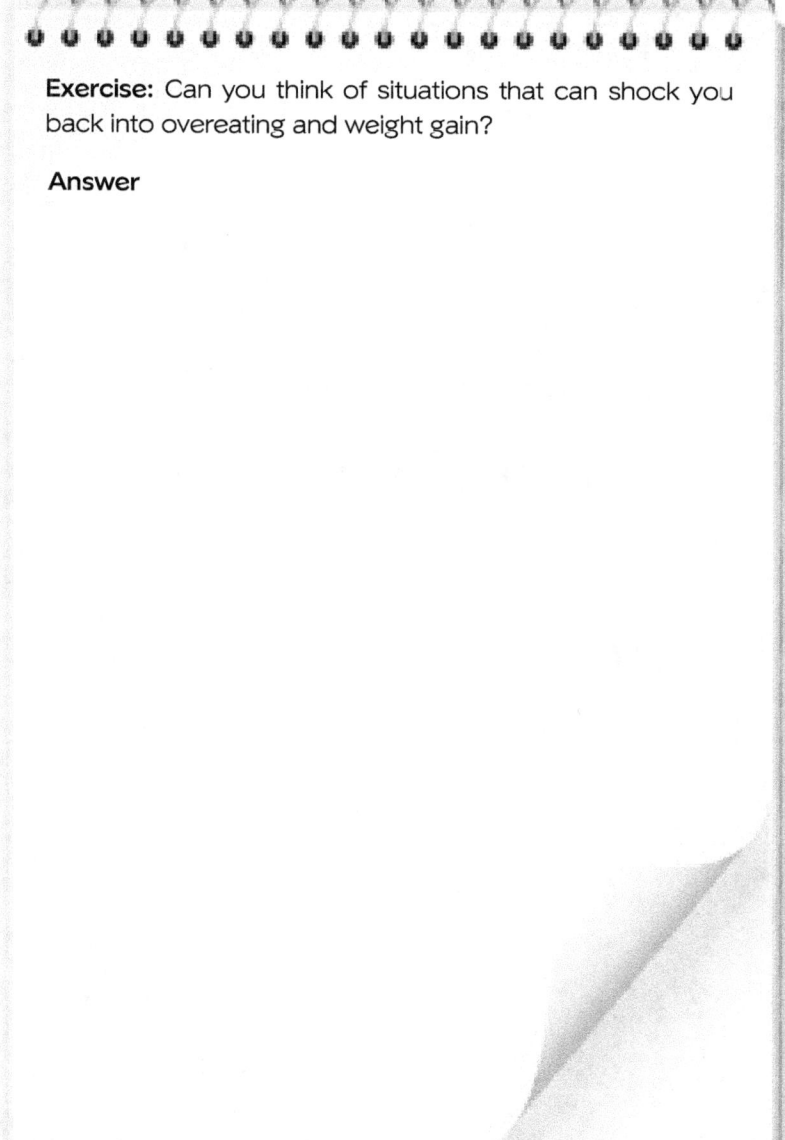

Exercise: Can you think of situations that can shock you back into overeating and weight gain?

Answer

Chapter Seven

Invest in Yourself

Think of your weight-loss efforts as a long-term investment. You will be getting a wonderful thing in return—a healthy and slim body you can enjoy every day. To arrive at your goal of having a healthy body, you should be prepared to invest and pay with your time, effort and, yes, some of your money.

I remember a story about one of my friends who was always talking about how he wished to lose weight and be his old slim self. He told me the usual story—that he had tried everything but with little or no success. I told him he was much too involved in work and wasn't focusing enough on his weight-loss efforts. I suggested that he take a vacation and go to a weight-loss retreat where he could focus on controlling food and have a program specifically tailored to him to engage in sports and other activities. He seemed to agree with my suggestion and told me he would take my advice and that he was just waiting for his annual leave. When his annual leave came, however, he had lost interest in the whole idea, and he told me very frankly, "I don't want to waste my leave days or money on a wellness retreat."

The point of this story is that many people want to lose weight but are not willing to spend anything on it—whether it be time, money or effort. When they are asked to make some sacrifices, weight loss goes down to the bottom of the priority list as compared to relaxing and earning money. And like my friend, some people think that such an investment in the tools to lose weight seems like a "waste."

In this chapter, I will provide some suggestions to expedite your weight loss. One of them includes going to a wellness retreat—this can have a "magical" impact on your weight loss goals, but you need to be prepared to spend quite a sum of money. And it's not just money that you need to part with, it can also be your free time or vacation days. We all love our time and money, but the thing is, you need to love the commitment to arrive at your desirable/healthy weight as much you love your other priorities in life.

You make many investments in your life. You invest time in teaching your children, hoping they will be successful later in life. You invest time in striking up friendships and maintaining them, hoping that you will not be left alone. You invest in your retirement fund to help you maintain your living standard even in your later years. If all these investments matter to you, then you need to top them with a desire to invest in your health—your body. This goes beyond just having a slim body so that you can walk confidently around the beach. It's a matter of being illness-free or not. Medical evidence on the correlation between diabetes and heart disease and being overweight just cannot be argued with. If you fail to maintain your health due in part to your weight and fall ill, then you will not be able to enjoy any of the returns on many of the investments you worked so dearly for.

Invest in Sports

You noticed in the 20% OFF program that I didn't include sports in the elements of the system. I did that for the following reasons:

1 To avoid distracting you. The reality in weight reduction is that if you want to lose weight, you need to work on controlling your food intake. For a majority of people, controlling what they eat is very tough, and they will be happy to start an exercise program to distract themselves from that reality. In my case, for example, I still remember my wife asking me: "How do you plan on reducing your weight when you keep eating the same amount of food?" My response was: "But I am playing sports, I will burn off all that food." However, if you read the "Educate Yourself" chapter in this book, you will know that sports alone are not enough to burn all that you eat, if you overeat. Eating a small candy bar will require you to take a long walk to burn off all the calories it contains (how about a 50-minute walk to burn the calories in a Snickers bar?). Sports are important for losing weight, but not as important as controlling food intake. So you should focus all your attention on the latter at the beginning of your eating program.

2 I want you to keep pursuing the 20% OFF program for as long as is necessary until you see some tangible results. I mentioned in the first part

of this book that the main reason people fail in their weight-loss efforts is due in fact to their not continuing with their diet long enough to see some tangible results that would encourage them to continue. But how will sports affect that? you might wonder. Well, when you play sports, your body will require more energy. Your body will not immediately go into a "fat storage mode," but rather will work on your appetite so that you eat more and take in food, like sugar-heavy "food," that provides quick bursts of energy. If you resist the hunger pangs, you will start feeling low in energy and might get headaches. What will happen later is that you will succumb to the urge to eat and, chances are, you will not eat only enough to cover the caloric requirements of your sporting activities, but will eat more than what you need, leading to unhealthy weight gain.

3   Change management and cycling. I found out that if you start with sports later in your program, you can use it as a break for any boredom that might set in while you're dieting. You can also assess how your body responds when you control food alone and when you control food plus exercise (in terms of losing weight). I discovered that I lose more weight when I focus on the 20% Off diet without engaging in any sports. This led me to the conclusion that, without sports, I actually have more energy to focus on the eating program. However, I have to engage in sports to maintain the weight loss I have achieved, especially during those times when I have not been following the 20% Off program fully.

You should not think, however, that, having said the above, I am downgrading the importance of sports in weight loss. On the contrary, exercising is very important, but you should just avoid it for the first few weeks until you start seeing results from your dieting.

Now let's shift to the importance of exercising. It is estimated that in order to lose one pound of weight, you need to burn a total of 3,600 additional calories. The good news is that you are always burning calories, even while you sleep. However, you burn very little during such periods of relative inactivity. For example, in a period of 30 minutes, you burn about 30 calories while you are sitting and watching TV, and about 160 while doing general gardening (that's not enough to burn the 270 calories in a normal-sized

Snickers bar). Compare this to sports, where you can burn more than 400 calories per hour in activities like running and cycling. However, note that these figures for the amount of calories burned depend on the intensity of the sport you are engaged in and your weight. Nevertheless, we can use them to shed light on how our body uses energy stored in food.

Exercising will help you burn more calories in less time, and it has many other bonuses. For example, you will be building muscles by exercising, and muscle tissue is found to burn more calories than any other tissue in your body. Another benefit is psychological, in that most people report an increase in "good feelings" while they are on an exercise program. This "feeling good" should help you be more optimistic about your weight-loss goals and feel that you can achieve exactly what you set out to do.

Experts advise that you should look for a sport you enjoy doing. That way, you will continue doing it without having to be reminded or pushed. However, I advise you to separate sports into two categories: the ones you enjoy, and the ones you need to do for weight loss. This might seem strange, but read on and you will see the logic behind my reasoning. The sport you like and the sport intended for your weight-loss goals can be the same thing, only IF they are activities like jogging or a variation of this, like brisk walking or running. Throughout my book, I have tried to be flexible and given you much room to implement this eating program based on your unique individual requirements (for instance, you can select your own method with which to shock yourself and the percentage of food you choose leave on the dish). For my part, I have found jogging to be the best sports activity if your desire is to lose weight and keep it off, based on the following reasons:

1 Jogging is not gimmick sport. Even the military use it to train their soldiers. This fact has kept me preoccupied for a long time—when someone joins the army, he/she starts by running as part of basic training. There certainly is something practical about this type of exercise.

2 You burn more calories when jogging or (better yet) running than if you engage in any other sport.

3   You get a huge "carryover" from jogging to your everyday life. You will feel lighter when you move, can keep up when playing with your children, and if the elevator to your apartment is not functional, you can easily use the stairs without needing to take the next day off from work (overkill, but I suppose you get the idea).

4   It's easy to learn, inexpensive and can be done alone or in the company of others.

5   You don't need special facilities or equipment to jog, just your shoes and a safe running path. So you don't have any excuses not to exercise.

6   You can use a treadmill if you can't go outdoors (especially during the rainy season). Treadmills have become very popular—with excellent reliability and features (like different programs and the ability to track your progress).

7   You never see a jogger or runner who is overweight.

In my case, I didn't immediately take up jogging. I liked lifting weights, and pretty much stuck with it. However, trying to lose weight by lifting weights just didn't do it. I had a strong feeling inside me that I needed to jog or run. I saw people jogging or running, and not a single one was overweight! Yet there I was, lifting weights with a big tummy jutting out in front of me. I suddenly felt determined to jog. It was like bitter medicine—I knew it would benefit me, but that it would also be difficult. And difficult it indeed was. I could not jog for more than 3 minutes without feeling my legs hurt. I even found it difficult to walk the next day when I got out of bed. However, in time, I grew to like jogging, and my running shoes became an essential item on my list of things to pack when I travel. I still lift weights sparingly, but I made it clear to myself that jogging is my choice of sport for losing weight (and maintaining it), and that any other sport would be for the enjoyment, challenge and purpose of socializing.

Before I go any further, I have to advise you that you need to see your doctor to be sure you can start on an exercise program. You should be particularly keen to know from your doctor whether your joints will be able to bear the impact of jogging, and whether your heart and lungs can function under the stress of strenuous sports activities.

Note that when I speak about jogging, you actually have 2 other options, either to walk briskly or run. However, for me, I found running to be very hard on my legs, whereas walking yielded few results and was somewhat boring.

You will find many books dedicated to a discussion on jogging, but this book is not one of those. However, I will provide some guidelines on how to embark on an excercise plan based on jogging, and I advise you to seek more information on the subject either from experts, from print sources or the Internet. To start on jogging, consider the following:

1   Start. If it took only becoming convinced about an idea to start on something, then all people would be achievers. It's not easy to just start jogging, though, especially when you have a career and a family that seem to take up so much of your time and energy. During my teenage years, I had nothing better to do than play sports or read and talk about books. However, now that I have my wife, kids, work and hobbies, things are a bit different. Now I have a big-screen TV and several laptops, and can afford a $7 cappuccino from the coffee shop. These things were all competing for my time: my laptop, TV and coffee. To start jogging, you need to flood your mind with thoughts that jogging is a must for your weight loss (or at least to keep the weight you lost from coming back).

2   Learn about jogging. When I first started out, I was able to jog for only about 3 minutes straight. If I forced myself to jog for 5 minutes, my legs and feet hurt badly the following day, to the point that I was unable to walk immediately when I got out of bed. However, I was convinced that jogging was the way to go, and I started to look at my jogging form. I discovered a wealth of information about foot types, shoes and heel striking. I found that using simple tips like how to space my feet and position my head could actually lessen the aching. Now I can jog for a full hour, and I do 3 miles daily with little or no soreness, something that I didn't think was possible before. You can educate yourself about jogging from the Internet, where you can find good instructional videos

at YouTube.com. However, a better solution is to join a running club if one is available in your area and seek the help of experts to guide you on how to improve your jogging.

3   Make a favorable association with jogging. What I mean is that you have to select something you like to do very much and then only do it while you jog. For example, I like to listen to audio books on my mp3 player. I took it upon myself not to listen to these books, though, unless I am on my treadmill. I even keep my mp3 player on the treadmill all the time. I then found myself very eager to use the treadmill so that I could listen to my audio books. This small trick contributed a lot to keeping me on the jogging track. You can make your own association. For example, you may want to put your treadmill in your living room and watch your favorite television program while exercising. Another good idea is to go jogging in your favorite park, or to use jogging as a means to meet with your friends instead of just going to the mall.

4   Push the priority of your jogging time. This is a technique I used when I first started jogging. Like most people, I had my 24 hours per day distributed among certain activities like work, sleep, family and watching TV. I was busy and couldn't imagine that I could dedicate time to jogging. What I did was, I forced the jogging time to take the place of other activities I liked doing. For instance, I liked to watch TV before going to bed, but now I was so actively thinking about jogging that if I didn't jog during my day, I would do it instead of watching TV even if it was late at night. I don't know if you can imagine yourself putting on your shoes and heading for the treadmill at 11:00 p.m. It was hard … very hard, but after the first 10 minutes, I was already feeling great. I basically sacrificed some of my choice activities for jogging, which sent a message to myself that I was really quite serious about my commitment to it. Little by little, jogging established itself as a daily activity, and I reached a point when, if I didn't jog for one day, I would feel that I had missed something really important.

5   Motivate yourself. Always set targets and work hard to exceed them. I like the words of Beverly Sills: "There are no shortcuts to any place

worth going." You need to start light and work your way up slowly. Set small targets and try to achieve them, and once you do, raise the bar a little bit higher. I have learned from life that if you keep doing something, chances are you will master it in time. I went from 3-minute jogs to jogging for 60 minutes. That's like a 2000% increase, but it didn't happen quickly. I increased the time gradually from 3 minutes to 10, 15, etc. I was very happy to be able to jog for 30 minutes, and I kept going till I reached 60 minutes, and I will keep on going. (Who knows? I might run a marathon!).

Under the same subject of motivation, I should warn you about being greedy. Chances are that in time, you will become a very good jogger or runner, but don't overdo it, else, you will burn yourself out. The term for doing too much sports is "overtraining," i.e. if you don't give yourself enough rest, you might cause injuries to your muscles and other tissues. Overtraining can also affect our feelings and cause unjustified boredom with a sport, which eventually leads to a person quitting exercising. So take it easy. Even when you become a really good jogger, take some days off, recharge and rest. My experience was that if I pushed myself too hard, I would stop jogging for periods of up to a full week due to aches and a really bad mood. I didn't want to risk quitting jogging, so I learned how to listen to my body and be aware of the times when excessive jogging might have negative results on what I had already achieved.

To summarize this section, I have advised you to play a particular sport for the specific purpose of weight loss, which is jogging. I have also advised you not to start exercising in the first few weeks of our eating program. Exercising is important and will help you feel good and maintain your weight, so make sure you invest in it.

Don't Go Cheap

I have another story for the many people who want to lose weight but are not willing to invest in that. I had a work colleague who was talking about buying a treadmill for so long and was convinced that having such equipment in his house would motivate him to exercise. One day, he called me after work to go looking for a treadmill. Despite my repeated advice to buy a good-quality treadmill, he bought one of the cheapest models. To put things into perspective, my co-worker had just bought a $70,000 Lexus a few weeks before this incident. Anyway, what I feared might happen did happen. He didn't enjoy the feel of the treadmill. "It's different from the ones in the gym," he told me, and like a lot of ill-bought exercise equipment around the world, the treadmill turned into an expensive clothes hanger.

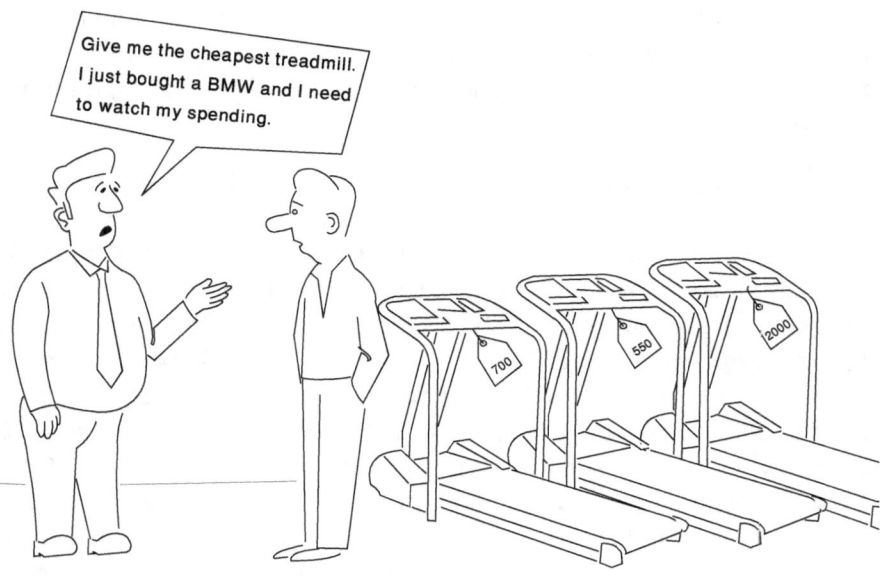

I am very vocal about buying good-quality exercise equipment, to a point that my friends feel they have to defend themselves and convince me that they are not cheap. I usually make them feel uncomfortable by my offers to provide the extra cash just so they can get a good-quality machine. I am not asking you to buy equipment that is for commercial use, like that used in gyms, but I want you to look for models that are on the borderline between home use and club use. I know equipment in this area is a bit expensive, but it's better than buying a piece of equipment you won't be able to use. Many people (including me) know about exercise equipment from gyms, and the story goes like this: we like one type of equipment in the gym, we use it every time we work out there, and feel we have found our dream machine. We reason that if we have this equipment in our house, we will cut the costs of memberships and will not need to buy fancy exercise clothing to impress others. We go shopping for that equipment, and it is very expensive. We go to a local store, find a similar piece of equipment and buy it, but "it doesn't feel like the one in the gym." We stop using it. As for myself, this story was repeated many times. I had exercise equipment from all different manufacturers and of all different types. I had a treadmill, home gym sets, an elliptical trainer, dumbbells and 3 different ab exercise machines. However, I didn't continue to use any single one of them. Actually, for some of the ab exercise machines, I used them only once—immediately after assembling them.

Finally, I started to think about the many pieces of exercise equipment I had and why I was not using them. I thought it was the atmosphere of the gym, where I could see people and people could see me, so I got motivated. But I was also able to exercise happily in times when there was no one else in the gyms I used. Maybe it was the feeling of heaviness, the quality and the smoothness of the gym equipment that I missed. For example, the treadmill I had at home cost me only $300, but it was small, narrow and noisy, and it shook under my pounding feet. It also lacked the many functions available on the gym treadmills, such as a heart monitor and a gauge for the different exercise levels. For these reasons, when I used my home treadmill, what I felt was akin to being removed from my first-class seat in an airplane, to an economy seat at the back. This feeling didn't make me want to use the treadmill, and it just sat there. Like I said, I had a lot of equipment … all of it with a price in the range of $50-$300. After doing the math, I figured out that their total cost amounted to more than $2000, which could have gotten me one pretty good treadmill. I also felt bad because I wasn't able to sell off the used equipment, so whenever I looked at it, I was reminded of my lost investment.

I eventually forced myself to buy a good treadmill, and gave away the other stuff that I owned. I felt happier because I used my money to buy a machine that I now use almost daily.

I urge you to do the same, and to spend your money on quality equipment that you believe in and like to use. If you take my advice to use jogging as the sport of choice to lose your excess weight, then go shopping for a treadmill (unless you jog outside) and search on the Internet for the equipment with the best prices and good customer satisfaction (feedback on products is available online too). You need to stay away from gimmicks and imitations. They will not only be a waste of your money, but might even affect your self-esteem, making you think you don't use them because you don't have willpower, and not because they are of low quality. Even if you decide to jog outside and don't need a treadmill, you should invest in your running gear and buy quality running shoes. This is the message I want to send in this section: Be prepared to spend on your weight loss goals, because in the end, it's all worth it.

Wellness Centers

I am an advocate of weight-loss vacations. These holidays almost certainly will help you achieve some weight-loss results that will motivate you to continue losing even more weight. Visiting wellness centers is becoming very popular, and I have visited many places like India, Thailand and the Czech Republic. Basically, you go on a trip to a hotel or resort that will control your food intake. These hotels and resorts are usually a little distance away from the main cities, so you don't have much choice in not following the food that will be prescribed/given to you. In addition, these places are usually packed with activities like sports, yoga, sightseeing, reading and massages, in the hope that these activities will distract you from the initial (but strong) discomfort associated with controlling (reducing) food intake. I have had very good experiences with such resorts, and I recommend them for the following reasons:

1   When going on a vacation for the sole purpose of losing weight, chances are you will be more committed to your goal (you will not want to go back home weighing the same after spending a lot of money; your mind will resist this and boost your commitment to reduce your weight).

2   The atmosphere in weight-loss centers is usually very relaxed and will also help you to de-stress yourself.

3 In these centers, staff are already experienced in dealing with overweight people and offer many remedies like serving tasty food that is low in calories and providing exercising programs.

4 Changing your external environment will help you change your thoughts and believe in nutrition and exercise. For example, when you are surrounded by people who are always conscious about food and sports, you will tend to join them in their thinking. In a sense, changing the outside can help change the inside.

5 You will have the chance to associate weight loss with fun things like meeting interesting people and visiting new places.

To find a weight-loss vacation center, you should do some research on the subject and read as many reviews as you can about different wellness centers. Use the Internet and search for terms like "wellness vacation," "weight-loss centers" and "weight-loss retreats." Also, check travel magazines for reviews. I have not included reviews in my book because I believe such information must be dynamic, and you should always look for the latest information available. Make sure to contact the wellness center you select and see what kind of services they offer. You should look for centers that have among their staff, doctors and/or nutritionists who specialize in weight management. In addition, look for centers that offer a balanced (and controlled) food plan that they will serve you and will ensure that you follow it.

Plan to stay for a reasonable length of time at the wellness center (I recommend at least 2 weeks), and make sure that the center has different activities on offer so you don't get bored.

I will close this chapter with a story of one of my friends who went to "Kalvory Vary" in the Czech Republic for a one-month weight-loss program. When he arrived, he was booked for an appointment with the center's physician, who did routine checks on my friend and said that he would be given balanced meals and controlled food intake and advised him to walk for 3 miles a day around the beautiful city. My friend was upset and told the doctor, "Well, I can do all that in my country, is this all that you can offer?" The doctor replied, "Actually, if you were able to do these simple things in your country, then you would not need to come here." It was a simple answer, but quite loaded with meaning. Weight loss is not very difficult in principle, but achieving it is a totally different thing. My friend continued with the vacation and came home weighing 15 pounds less.

Quality of Food

Let's face it, good food is not cheap. It's not that it's so expensive, but junk food, which is quite abundant, is so much cheaper. For the purpose of weight loss, "good" food is USUALLY better in terms of having less calories and the absence of fat and added sugar. Consider the difference in price between a loaf of wheat bread and white bread, or between a double cheeseburger and a grilled chicken burger. Food high in calories is usually more convenient to eat, e.g. how about eating canned pineapple vs. peeling and slicing a fresh version of the fruit?

You need to be prepared to adjust your grocery-shopping budget, which might get a little bit higher because of your new food selections. When I became more conscious about my food shopping, I faced many difficulties. For example, it was hard for me to buy wheat bread at almost double the price of white bread (also, white bread tasted better). However, my only relief was the thought that I had to invest in my weight-loss goals, and that if I wanted a better body, I needed to be ready to pay for it. The good news is that things (with your money expenditure) will settle down. With time and conscious thinking between alternatives, you will be able to find ways to compensate for the increase in the cost of your food shopping by buying less chocolate, sweets and cakes, or even cutting down on other expensive merchandise like clothing.

Final Statement

Losing weight is not a one-time competition that you need to win and then forget about it. It is a life-long commitment. If I could go back in time, I would make sure I never woke up the fat man inside me, but it's too late for me. I spent a lot of money and effort to lose weight, but in return, I am full of happiness and satisfaction that words cannot describe. It's not a mere dream that turned real, but rather a fantasy that became a reality.

I hope that I was able in this book to share my experience with you and suggest a program that will help you take real steps toward losing weight. I hope that you stop viewing weight loss as a matter of only willpower, and please stop blaming overweight people as being weak and undisciplined. It's very hard for them, and no one can understand their suffering unless he/she experiences what they live through every day.

Take extra care of your kids. Teach them to make good food choices and to enjoy eating healthy food. I teach them that it's OK not to finish their dish as long as they feel full. I will do all my best so that they do not experience what it feels like to be an obese person.

I would be very happy to hear from you, so please visit this book website at www.20offdiet.com and share any comments or suggestions you have.

www.ingramcontent.com/pod-product-compliance
Lightning Source LLC
Chambersburg PA
CBHW072131280526
45788CB00002B/590